ACTIVATE YOUR BRAIN

Brain Training, Strategies to Learn Faster and Better and Obtain Mental Flexibility, Concentration and Meditation, Clean Your Mind and Make it Unlimited

Richard L Bolton

© Copyright 2020 By Richard L Bolton
All rights reserved.

This document is geared towards providing exact and reliable information with regards to the topic and issue covered. The publication is sold with the idea that the publisher is not required to render accounting, officially permitted, or otherwise, qualified services. If advice is necessary, legal or professional, a practiced individual in the profession should be ordered.

From a Declaration of Principles which was accepted and approved equally by a Committee of the American Bar Association and a Committee of Publishers and Associations.

In no way is it legal to reproduce, duplicate, or transmit any part of this document in either electronic means or in printed format. Recording of this publication is strictly prohibited and any storage of this document is not allowed unless with written permission from the publisher. All rights reserved.

The information provided herein is stated to be truthful and consistent, in that any liability, in terms of inattention or otherwise, by any usage or abuse of any policies, processes, or directions contained within is the solitary and utter responsibility of the recipient reader. Under no circumstances will any legal responsibility or blame be held against the publisher for any reparation, damages, or monetary loss due to the information herein, either directly or indirectly.

Respective authors own all copyrights not held by the publisher.

The information herein is offered for informational purposes solely, and is universal as so. The presentation of the information is without contract or any type of guarantee assurance.

The trademarks that are used are without any consent, and the publication of the trademark is without permission or backing by the trademark owner. All trademarks and brands within this book are for clarifying purposes only and are the owned by the owners themselves, not affiliated with this document.

TABLE OF CONTENTS

INTRODUCTION

The Advancement of Our Brain From its Beginning in Ancient Seas to its Significant Expansion.

The tale of the brain starts in the old seas, long before the initial animals appeared. The single-celled organisms that crawled or swam in them might not have had minds. However, they did have sophisticated methods of noticing and responding to their setting.

"These devices are maintained right through to the evolution of mammals," states Seth Give at the Wellcome Count On Sanger Institute in Cambridge, UK. "That's a deep ancestry."

The evolution of multicellular pets depended on cells being able to feel as well as react to other cells-- to interact. For instance, Sponges filter their food from the water they pump via the channels in their bodies.

 They can gradually inflate as well as tighten these networks to get rid of any sediment and also avoid them clogging up.

These activities are triggered when cells identify chemical messengers like glutamate or GABA, pumped out by various other cells in the sponge. These chemicals play a comparable duty in our brains today.

Deploying any chemicals into the water is a very sluggish way of interacting with far-off cells-- it can take a great few mins for a demosponge to pump up and also close its networks.

 Glass sponges have a faster way: they fire an electric pulse across their body that makes all the flagella that pump water with their bodies quit within a matter of secs.

This is feasible since all living cells generate an electric possible across their membranes by draining ions, opening up networks that allow ions stream freely throughout the membrane layer creates sudden changes in this possibility.

 If neighboring ion channels likewise open in response, a sort of Mexican wave can travel along a cell's surface area at rates of several meters a second. Because the cells in glass sponges are integrated, these impulses can take a trip across their whole bodies.

Deep origins

on to various other cells by releasing chemicals such as glutamate, yet they do so where they meet them, at Recent studies have revealed that a lot of the elements needed to transfer electric signals, as well as to launch and. Find chemical signals, are located in single-celled micro-organisms referred to as choanoflagellates.

That is significant since old choanoflagellates are believed to have triggered pets around 850 million years ago.

So almost from the beginning, the cells within very first pets had the potential to interact with each other using electrical chemical signals and pulses. It wasn't a big leap for some cells to end up being experts for lugging messages.

These nerve cells evolved long, wire-like expansions-- axons-- for carrying electric signals over long distances. They still pass signals synapses. That means the chemicals only need to diffuse throughout a tiny void, substantially speeding points up. And so, really beforehand, the nervous system was born.

The first neurons were possibly connected, in a scattered network throughout the body (see layout). This sort of structure, called a nerve web, can still be seen in the quivering collections of jellyfish and sea anemone.

Yet in other pets, groups of neurons began to show up-- a central nervous system. These permitted the information to be processed rather than merely communicated, allowing animals to move and also reply to the environment in every other innovative way.

The most specific teams of the nerve cells are the first brain-like framework-- established near the mouth and also primitive eyes.

Our view of this momentous occasion is hazy. According to lots of biologists, it occurred in a worm-like creature called the urbilaterian (see layout), the ancestor of the majority of living pets including vertebrates, mollusks, and. Also, pests Oddly, though, a few of its offspring, such as the acorn worm, lack this neuronal hub.

There is a possibility that the urbilaterian never had a mind, which, later on, evolved on its own. Or it could be that the progenitor of the acorn worm had a primitive brain and lost it-- which suggests the prices of structure minds sometimes surpass the advantages.

Regardless, a central, brain-like framework existed in the forefathers of the animals. These primitive, fish-like creatures most likely appeared like the living lancelet, a jawless filter-feeder.

The mind of the lancelet barely stands out from the remainder of the spinal cord, yet was experts regions are apparent: the hindbrain manages its swimming skill, as an example, while its forebrain is apart of the innovation.

"They are to vertebrates that which a small country church is to Notre Dame cathedral-- the basic architecture is there though they lack a great deal of the complexity," says Linda Holland at the College of California, San Diego.

There are some fish-like filter feeders required to connect their body to rocks. Swimming larvae of sea squirts have a relaxed brain once they settle down on a rock it deteriorates and is soaked up right into the body.

We would not be below, naturally, if our ancestors had not maintained swimming. And also around 500 million years ago, points went wrong when among them was recreating, causing its entire genome obtaining copied. This, however, happened not just once, two times.

These crashes led the way for the evolution of even more facility minds by supplying a lot of spare genetics that can evolve in different directions as well as handle brand-new roles.

"It resembles the moment your parents purchased you the greatest Lego package-- with lots of different parts to use in various combinations," states Grant.

Among lots of various other points, it allowed different mind regions to share various sorts of natural chemicals, which in turn allowed much more cutting-edge habits to arise.

As early fish battled to find food as well as friends, and dodge killers, a lot of the core structures still discovered in our minds developed.

The optic tectum is associated with tracking. Relocates items with the eyes; the amygdala, which helps us to reply to afraid situations; parts of the limbic system, which offers us our sensations of incentive as well as helps to put down memories; and the basal ganglia, which manage patterns of activities.

Brainy animals

By 360 million years back, our ancestors had colonized the land, eventually triggering the very first animals about 200 million years earlier.
These creatures already had a small neocortex-- added layers of neural tissue externally of the mind responsible for the intricacy and also versatility of animal behavior. As well as when did this critical area evolve? That stays an enigma.
Living reptiles amphibians and do not have a straight equivalent, and since their minds do not load their entire head cavity, fossils inform us little regarding the souls of our amphibian and reptilian forefathers.
The fact is that the brain size of animals boosted relative to their bodies as they struggled to contend with the dinosaurs. By this point, the brain loaded the head, leaving impressions that provide telltale indications of the changes that bring about this neural expansion.
Timothy Rowe at the College of Texas at Austin lately used CT scans to check out the brain dental caries of fossils of two very early mammal-like pets, Morganucodon and also Hadrocodium, both tiny, shrew-like creatures that fed on bugs.
This type of research study has just lately come to be possible. "You might hold these fossils in your hands as well as recognize that they have solutions about the development of the brain. However, there was no other way to enter them non-destructively," he claims. "It's only now that we can get in their heads.".
Rowe's scans exposed that the first considerable rises in dimension were in the olfactory bulb, suggesting creatures pertained to depend significantly on their noses to seek food. There were also significant increases approximately the neocortex that map tactile sensations-- most likely the ruffling of hair in particular—
which suggests the sense of touch was crucial as well the searching for suit perfectly with the commonly held concept that very early animals were nocturnal, hiding throughout the day as well as scampering about in the hedge in the evening when less hungry dinosaurs were running around.
After the dinosaurs were wiped out, in about 65 million years back, a few of the animals that made it through took to the trees-- the ancestors of the primates.
Good sight helped them go after bugs around trees, which caused an expansion of the visual part of the neocortex. The most significant

psychological challenge, however, may have been keeping track of their social lives.

If modern primates are anything to pass, their ancestors likely stayed in teams. Mastering the social niceties of team living needs a great deal of brainpower.

Robin Dunbar at the College of Oxford assumes this could describe the massive growth of the frontal areas of the primate neocortex, especially in the apes. "You need extra calculating power to handle those partnerships," he states.

Dunbar has shown there is a strong partnership between the size of primate groups, the regularity of their interactions with each other as well as the size of the frontal neocortex in numerous varieties.

Besides boosting in size, these frontal areas additionally progressed linked, both within themselves, as well as to various other parts of the mind that take care of sensory input and also electric motor control.

Such changes can also be seen in the specific neurons within these regions, which have advanced extra input and outcome factors.

All of which geared up the later primates with a remarkable ability to incorporate as well as refine the info reaching their bodies, and then regulate their actions based upon this sort of deliberative reasoning.

Besides raising their total knowledge, this eventually results in some abstract thought: the extra the brain refines incoming details, the much more it starts to recognize and also look for overarching patterns that are a step away from the concrete, physical things before the eyes which brings us nicely to an ape that lived regarding 14 million years earlier in African countries.

It was a very smart ape; in other words, the brains of almost all of its descendants-- orang-utans, gorillas, and also primates do not appear to have significantly transformed compared with the branch of its household that led to us. What made us various?

We most times believe that moving out of the forests and taking to strolling on two legs cause the expansion of our minds. Fossil explorations, nonetheless, show that millions of years after early hominids became bipedal, they still had little brains.

We can only speculate about why their minds began to grow bigger around 2.5 million years ago, but it is feasible that luck figured in.

In other primates, the "attack" muscle exerts a potent force across the whole of the skull, constricting its growth. In our forefathers, this muscle mass was deteriorated by a single mutation, perhaps breaking the ice for the head to increase.

This mutation occurred around the very same time as the first humans with weaker jaws and bigger skulls, and also brains appeared.

Once we got clever sufficient to introduce and take on smarter lifestyles, the impact of a positive comment might have started, resulting in more brain expansion.

"If you desire a huge brain, you have reached feed it," mentions Todd Preuss of Emory University in Atlanta, Georgia.

He assumes the advancement of tools to kill and also butcher animals around 2 million years earlier would have been essential for the expansion of the human mind, because the meat is such an abundant source of nutrients.

A more prosperous diet plan, consequently, would have opened the door to further brain growth. Primatologist Richard Wrangham at Harvard University believes that fire played a comparable role by permitting us to obtain even more nutrients from our food.

Consuming prepared food resulted in the diminishing of our intestines, he recommends. Because gut tissue is pricey to grow and also preserve, this loss would have liberated priceless resources, once more favoring further mind development.

Mathematical versions by Luke Rendell as well as coworkers at the College of St Andrews in the UK not only back the suggestion that cultural and genetic evolution can feed off each other, they recommend this can generate extreme selection pressures that result in "runaway" development of specific qualities.

This type of feedback may have played a significant role in our language abilities. As soon as early people started speaking, there would undoubtedly be a reliable option for anomalies that enhanced this ability, such as the famous FOXP2 gene, which makes it possible for the basal ganglia and the cerebellum to put down the complicated motor memories necessary for complex speech.

" Social and genetic development can feed off each other, leading to 'runaway' evolution."

The general image is one of a virtuous cycle involving our diet regimen, society, modern technology, social connections as well as genetics. It resulted in the contemporary human mind coming into existence in Africa by about 200,000 years back.

Development never stops, however. According to one recent research, the visual cortex ha grown larger in individuals that migrated from Africa to northern latitudes, possibly to aid offset the dimmer brighten there.

Downhill from here

So why didn't our brains get even bigger? It may be because we reached a factor at which the benefits of larger brains began to be surpassed by the dangers of bringing to life kids with big heads. Or it could have been an instance of diminishing returns.

Our brains are instead starving, melting 20 percent of our food at a price of about 15 watts, and any type of additional improvements would undoubtedly be significantly demanding. Simon Laughlin at the College of Cambridge contrasts the mind to a sports car, which melts ever before a lot more fuel the much faster it goes.

One way to speed up our brain, as an example, would be to advance nerve cells that can discharge even more times per second.

Yet to support a 10-fold boost in the "clock rate" of our nerve cells, our mind would require to melt power at the very same price as Usain Screw's legs throughout a 100-meter sprint. The 10,000-calorie-a-day diet regimen of Olympic swimmer Michael Phelps would undoubtedly pale in comparison.

Not just did the development in the dimension of our minds stop around 200,000 years ago, in the past 10,000 to 15,000 years, the average size of the human brain compared with our body has diminished by 3 or 4 percent. Some see this as no cause for worry. Dimension, besides, isn't every little thing, as well as it's entirely feasible that the brain has just evolved to make better use much less grey and white issue.

 That would seem to fit with some hereditary researches, which recommends that our mind's circuitry is a lot more efficient now than it remained in the past." In the past 10,000 years, the typical dimension of the human brain has diminished".

Others, nonetheless, believe this shrinkage is a sign of a small decline in our necessary mental abilities.

 David Geary at the College of Missouri-Columbia, for one, thinks that when complex societies established, the less intelligent can survive on the backs of their smarter peers, whereas in the past, they would have passed away-- or a minimum of stopped working to discover a companion.

This decline might well be proceeding. Several research studies have located that the lot more intelligent individuals are, the fewer youngsters they tend to have.

 More than ever previously, intellectual as well as economic success are not linked with having a larger family. If it were, states Rendell, "Bill Gates would certainly have 500 kids.".

This evolutionary result would lead to a decline of about 0.8 IQ points per generation in the US if you exclude the effects of migration, a 2010 study wrapped up.

However, support issues in addition to nature: even if this genetic effect is real, it has been higher than made up for by enhanced healthcare and also education and learning, which led to a steady surge in INTELLIGENCE throughout most of the 20th century.

Crystal-ball gazing is always a danger, as well as we have no chance of recognizing the obstacles that humankind will deal with over the next centuries.

 However, if they transform whatsoever, it appears likely that our minds are going keep "declining"-- unless, indeed, we step in and take charge.

The feathery apes

Would certainly intelligent dinosaurs rule the world if a meteorite influence had not erased their kind?

We can not address that inquiry; however, there is no doubt that dinosaurs had the potential to advance into brilliant animals. The proof is sitting in a tree near you.

Particular birds, particularly the crow family members, have advanced difficult habits that match the ingenuity of several primates.

 Device use, deceptiveness, face recognition-- you call it, they can do it.

 Why are some birds so smart? Stig Walsh at the National Museums Scotland believes that structures were laid in their dinosaur ancestors, which most likely climbed up around in trees before eventually taking off.

 These actions would certainly have favored the same capabilities that developed in the tree-climbing primates: superb vision, electric motor control, and equilibrium, which came about through the growth of the mind locations called the optic tectum and the brain.

In other to take on various other animals, these tree-climbing dinosaurs could have likewise begun to progress new foraging approaches that required a lot more brainpower, causing the growth of the forebrain. There are lots of fossils of dinosaurs, he claims, whose minds already possess a few of these enlarged structures.

So the ancestors of birds had reasonably healthy minds compared with their body dimension, as well as their minds expanded proportionately also more prominent once they took off and progressed much more advanced practices.

 These capabilities may have allowed them to make it through the mass extinction that eliminated the other dinosaurs, Walsh says, considering that their ingenuity would undoubtedly have helped them to locate new methods of foraging for food following the catastrophe.

Bird brains can be structured in very various means to mammalian one s. The mammalian family tree developed brand-new external layers, known as the neocortex, which birds do not have. In spite of this, it is most likely that the enlarged frontal cortex of the animals, and the bigger forebrain of the birds, perform similar functions.

"There's been a merging, along with different courses," states Walsh. How wise could birds get? For all the tool-making talents of crows, a beak is not as helpful for adjusting things like the hands of primates. That might limit the growth of bird brains, though some have speculated that the wings of ground-living birds could yet re-evolve grasping forelimbs.

How Does The Brain Work?

The mind can function as a vast computer. It refines information that it receives from the detects and body, and sends out messages back to the body.

 Yet the mind can do a lot more than the equipment can: humans assume and also experience feelings with their brain, and also, it is the origin of human intelligence.

The human brain is approximately the dimension of 2 clenched fists and also considers concerning 1.5 kilos. From the outer part, it looks a little bit like a large walnut, with folds as well as gaps.

The mind cells are said to comprise of about 100 billion afferent neurons (nerve cells) as well as one trillion supporting cells that stabilize the cells.

There are various sections of the mind, each with their features:

- the cerebrum.
- the diencephalon-- including the thalamus, hypothalamus, and also pituitary gland.
- the mind stem-- including the midbrain, pons, and medulla.
- the brain.

Framework Of The Brain

The cerebrum has a right fifty percent and a left half, called the right and left hemispheres. Both hemispheres attach through a full package of nerve fibers called the corpus callosum.

Each hemisphere is composed of 6 locations (lobes) that have various features. The brain regulates activity as well as processes sensory details. Mindful and also unconscious actions and also sensations are produced below. It is likewise responsible for speech, hearing, knowledge, and memory.

The functions of both hemispheres are to a terrific degree various: whereas the left hemisphere is accountable for speech and abstract thinking in many people, the ideal region is usually in charge of spatial reasoning or imagery.

The right side of the mind controls the left side of the body, as well as the left side of the brain, which manages the appropriate team of the body.

The effect suggests that damage to the left hemisphere due to a stroke, for instance, can bring about paralysis on the right side of the body.

The left cerebral cortex is accountable for speech as well as language. The ideal cortex supplies spatial info, such as where your foot goes to the moment. The thalamus provides the brain with sensory info from the skin, eyes, and ears, along with other details.

The hypothalamus manages points like cravings, thirst as well as sleep. Along with the pituitary gland, it additionally manages the hormonal agents in your body.

The brain stem communicates details between the brain, the cerebellum, and also the spinal cord, as well as managing eye activities and even faces. It also controls essential features like breathing, high blood pressure, and heartbeat.

The brain collaborates movements as well as is accountable for the balance.

Just how Is The Brain Provided With Blood

The mind needs a steady flow of adequate oxygen, sugar, and also other nutrients. For that reason, it has a specifically good blood supply. Each side of the brain gets blood via three arteries:
- In the front, the former cerebral artery supplies the cells behind the forehead as well as under the crown (the top of the head).
- The middle cerebral artery is necessary for the sides and locations that are more inside the mind. The former and also center cerebral artery split off from the internal carotid artery, a significant blood vessel in the neck.
- The posterior cerebral artery provides the rear of the head, the lower part of the mind, as well as the cerebellum. The cerebellum is supplied with blood from the vertebral arteries, which are also significant arteries of the neck.
Before the three arteries get to "their" brain region, where they divided into smaller sized branches, they are close together listed below the brain. In this area, they are attached to every various other by smaller sized capillary-- forming a structure similar to a traffic circle. The arteries are attached per other in other views too. The advantage of these connections pose is that blood supply troubles in the brain can be compensated for somewhat:
As an example, if a branch of an artery progressively comes to be narrower, blood can still move to the part of the brain it provides through these alternative routes (security blood circulation).
The tiniest branches (blood vessels) of the arteries in the brain supply the mind cells with oxygen as well as nutrients from the blood-- but they do not allow various other materials to pass as conveniently as similar capillaries in the rest of the body do.
The clinical term for this sensation is the "blood-brain obstacle." It can secure the fragile brain from poisonous materials in the blood, as an example.
After oxygen has entered the cells, the oxygen-poor blood flows away through the veins of the brain (cerebral blood vessels). The seams lug the blood to larger capillary called sinuses.

The sinus wall surfaces are enhanced by a tough membrane layer (dura mater), which helps them keep their form too. This layer maintains them permanently open as well as makes it simple for the blood to move into the blood vessels in the neck.

Composition of the Brain

The brain serves many vital features. It provides meaning to things that occur in the world bordering us. With the five detects of sight, scent, hearing, touch as well as preference, the mind obtains messages, commonly lots of at the same time.

The mind manages thoughts, memory and speech, limb movements, and the feature of several organs within the body. It additionally accurately establishes how individuals respond to stressful circumstances (i.e., writing of a test, loss of a task, birth of a kid, ailment, etc.) by regulating heart as well as breathing prices. The mind is an arranged structure, split into lots of elements that serve details and vital features.

The weight of the brain changes its form from birth through adulthood. At birth, the typical brain considers one pound, as well as expands to concerning two pounds during childhood. The average weight of a grown-up female mind is about 2.7 pounds, while the mind of an adult male considers three extra pounds.

The Nerve system

The nerves are commonly divided into the central nerves and also the peripheral nervous system. The primary jumpy system is comprised of the brain, its cranial nerves, and the spine. The peripheral nervous system consists of the spinal nerves that branch from the spine and also the autonomous nerves (split right into the supportive and parasympathetic nerves).

The Cell Framework of the Mind

The mind is composed of 2 kinds of cells: nerve cells and also glial cells, additionally. Referred to as neuroglia or glia. The nerve cell is accountable for sending and getting nerve signals or impulses. Glial cells are non-neuronal cells that support, provide and also nourishment, keep homeostasis, type myelin, and promote signal transmission in the nerves. In the human brain, glial cells outnumber nerve cells by about 50 to one. Glial cells are the most normal cells located in essential mind tumors.

When a person is identified with a brain lump, a biopsy may be done, in which tissue is gotten rid of from the piece for recognition functions by a pathologist. Pathologists determine the type of cells that exist in this mind tissue, as well as brain tumors, are called based upon this organization. The sort of brain lump and also batteries included individual effect diagnosis as well as cure.

Meningeal

The brain which, is enclosed inside the bony covering called the skull. The skull protects the mind from injury. With each other, the skull and also bones that protect the face are called the head.

In between the skull and also the brain is meningeal, which consists of three layers of tissue that cover and also safeguard the brain as well as the spinal cord.

From the outer layer, inward are the arachnoid, pia mater, and tentorium meninx dura meninges.

Tentorium meninx dura: In the brain, the dura mater is made up of two layers of a whitish, nonelastic movie, or membrane layer. The external layer is called the periosteum. An internal covering, the dura, lines within the whole head and also creates little folds or areas in which parts of the mind are safeguarded and safeguarded.

Both unique folds up of the dura in mind are called the falx as well as the tentorium. The falx separates the right as well as the left half of the mind as well as the tentorium separates the top as well as the lower side of the brain.

Arachnoid: The other layer of the meningeal is the arachnoid. This membrane is thin and also fragile and also covers the whole mind. There is a room between the dura, and also the arachnoid membranes called the subdural area. The arachnoid consists of delicate, elastic tissue and even blood vessels of differing dimensions.

Pia Mater: The layer of meningeal closest to the outer area of the mind is called the pia mater. The pia mater has lots of capillaries that get to deep right into the surface area of the brain.

The pia, which covers the whole surface area of the brain, complies with the folds up of the brain. The significant arteries providing the brain provide the pia with its blood vessels.

The area that separates the arachnoid and the pia is called the sub-arachnoid area. It is within this location that cerebrospinal liquid flows.

Cerebrospinal Fluid
Cerebrospinal fluid (CSF) is discovered within the brain as well as surrounds the brain as well as the spine. Cerebrospinal fluid is a clear, watery substance that helps to support the mind as well as the spinal cord from injury. This fluid flows with networks around the spinal cord and brain, continually being taken in and also restored. It is within hollow fibers in the brain, called ventricles, where the liquid is generated.
A highly specialized structure within each ventricle, called the choroid plexus, is in charge of most of CSF manufacturing. The mind generally maintains a balance between the amount of CSF soaked up as well as the quantity is formed. Nonetheless, disruptions in this system may take place.

Ventricular System
The ventricular system is classed into four cavities called ventricles, which are connected by a series of holes, called foramen, and also tubes.

Two ventricles confined in the analytical hemispheres are called the side ventricles (first and also second). They each interact with the third ventricle with a separate opening called the Foramen of Munro. The 3rd ventricle remains in the center of the brain, and its walls are comprised of the thalamus and also hypothalamus.

The third ventricle gets in touch with the 4th ventricle through a long tube called the Aqueduct of Sylvius.

Brain Components and Features
Brainstem
The brainstem is the lower expansion of the brain, situated in front of the cerebellum and linked to the spinal cord. It contains three structures: the midbrain, pons, and also medulla oblongata. It works as a relay terminal, passing messages back and forth between different parts

of the body and the cortex. Numerous essential or primitive functions that are crucial for survival are found there.

The midbrain is an essential center for ocular movement while the pons is involved with coordinating eye and face activities, facial sensation, hearing, and also balance.

The medulla oblongata regulates breathing, blood pressure, heart rhythms, and also swallowing. Messages from the cortex to the nerves, spinal cord, and even that branch from the spine are sent out through the pons and also the brainstem. The devastation of these areas of the brain will undoubtedly cause "brain death." Without these vital functions, people can not survive.

The complicated triggering system is discovered in the midbrain, pons, medulla, and part of the thalamus. It controls levels of wakefulness, allows people to take note of their atmospheres as well as is associated with rest patterns.

Coming from the brainstem are 10 of the 12 cranial nerves that regulate hearing, eye activity, facial feelings, taste, ingesting as well as events of the face, neck, shoulder as well as tongue muscles. The cranial nerves for smell as well as vision come from the brain. Four sets of cranial nerves originate from the pons.

Cerebellum
The brain is located at the rear of the brain underneath the occipital wattles. It is divided from the cerebrum by the tentorium (layer of dura). The brain fine-tunes motor task or motion, e.g., the great movements of fingers as they perform the surgical treatment or suggest. It helps one preserve posture, sense of balance or equilibrium, by regulating the tone of muscles and the setting of limbs.
 The cerebellum is crucial in one's capability to carry out fast and also repetitive actions such as playing a computer game. In the brain, right-sided abnormalities create symptoms on the same side of the body.

Cerebrum

The cerebrum, which forms the major part of the mind, is split right into two huge parts: the right and also left analytical hemispheres. The brain is a term typically made use of to describe the whole brain. A fissure or groove that splits the two regions is called the terrific longitudinal crack. The two sides of the brain are signed up at the bottom by the corpus callosum.

The corpus callosum attaches the two fifty percent of the mind as well as delivers messages from one half of the brain to the various other. The surface of the cerebrum has billions of neurons as well as glia that, with each other, developing the layer.

The cerebral layer appears grayish-brown in color and is called the "gray matter." The surface of the brain appears wrinkled. The cortex has sulci (small grooves), cracks (larger grooves), as well as bulges in between the grooves, called gyri. Scientists have specific names for the bumps as well as slots on the surface of the brain.

Years of scientific study have exposed the specific features of the numerous regions of the brain. Under the cerebral cortex or surface of the brain, attaching fibers between nerve cells create a white-colored area called the "white matter."

The cerebral hemispheres have several distinctive fissures. By situating these landmarks externally of the brain, it can rightly be divided into sets of "lobes." Lobes are merely broad regions of the mind. The brain or brain can be split into pairs of frontal, temporal, parietal as well as occipital wattles. Each area has a frontal, temporal, parietal, and occipital wattle. Each lobe may be separated, once again, into locations that serve very certain features. The portions of the mind do not work alone: they function through very complex connections with one another.

Messages within the brain are provided in many means. The signals are transferred along with courses called pathways. Any devastation of brain cells by growth can interrupt the communication between various parts of the mind. The outcome will be a loss of function such as speech, the capacity to read, or the capability to comply with accessible spoken commands.

Messages can take a trip from one lump on the brain to another (gyri to gyri), from one wattle to another, from one side of the mind to the various other, from one lobe of the brain to structures that are located in the inner part the brain, e.g., thalamus, or from the deep structures of the brain to one more area in the central nerves.

Research study has determined that touching one side of the mind sends out electric signals to the opposite side of the body. Touching the electrical motor area on the appropriate side of the brain would undoubtedly cause the contrary side or the left side of the body to move. Boosting the left crucial motor cortex would undoubtedly create the ideal side of the body to move.
 The messages for activity and experience go across to the opposite side of the brain as well as cause the contrary arm or leg to relocate or feel an experience. The ideal side of the brain manages the left side of the body as well as the other way around. So if a brain growth occurs on the right side of the mind that regulates the movement of the arm, the left arm might be weak or paralyzed.

Cranial Nerves
Twelve pairs of nerves originate from the brain itself. These nerves are in charge of extremely details activities as well as its name as well as the phoned number as follows:

Olfactory: Odor
Optic: Visual fields as well as capacity to see
Oculomotor: Eye activities; eyelid opening
Trochlear: Eye activities
Trigeminal: Facial experience
Abducens: Eye activities
Facial: Eyelid closing; facial expression; taste sensation
Auditory/vestibular: Hearing; the sense of equilibrium
Glossopharyngeal: Preference experience; swallowing
Vagus: Ingesting; preference sensation
Accessory: Control of neck and shoulder muscles.

Peripheral nervous system advancement

The bilaterian nerves are subdivided into two main elements: the central as well as the peripheral nervous systems (CNS as well as PNS). Permanent cross-talk between the CNS as well as PNS is essential for the integration of sensory inputs.

In the fourth century BC, Alcmaeon of Croton recommended the initial theory about networks (" poroi" in old greek) that would attach the detects as well as the brain, this last one being the facility of human understanding. Later, it became clear that all sensory knowledge being mechanical, acoustic, gustatory, as well as olfactory were passed on to the CNS via the "nerve. Indeed, the precise interplay between these two networks established in parallel throughout embryonic growth.

Also, it has been demonstrated that both axon guidance and the neuronal task can actively regulate links between the PNS and also the CNS. Nevertheless, the PNS is itself created by various elements, each focused on the transmission of a particular signal to the CNS. These signals are transferred by mechanosensory, chemical, or thermal receptors predicting to the mammalian spinal cord via nociceptive afferents. Drosophila bristles are sensory organs that are snugly distributed as well as include one single mechanosensory nerve cell that particularly forecasts to the CNS. These axons can be assisted by cell adhesion molecules, such as Neuroglian or Flamingo, but also by various other advice particles, such as Plexins or semaphorins.

Down syndrome cell attachment molecule (DSCAM) is a transmembrane receptor of the immunoglobulin superfamily. DSCAM has since been defined to regulate cell targeting, axon branch spec, and dendrite pattern. The repulsive molecule, Slit, has been shown to bind and also signal through DSCAM1 individually of Robo receptors. Indeed, regional binding to Slit drives the spatial uniqueness of axon collateral formation.

Additionally, record that several DSCAM isoforms exist, and also particular DSCAM isoform mosaicism in a specific development cone appears to determine regional support decisions, such as the formation of axon collateral projections.

The internal ear is vital for the transmission of audios and also their assimilation by the CNS. This complex sensory body organ is made up of bipolar spiral ganglion nerve cells (SGN) that attach the ipsilateral cochlear nucleus and the mechanosensory inner and also outer hair cells located in the body organ of Corti.

SGNs project to both the internal (IHC) as well as the outer hair cells (OHC). During the program of growth, both kind I as well as II job to the OHC, but the type I SGNs show up to refine in later stages and also the only project to the IHC.

Making use of molecular pens to target solitary spiral ganglia has revealed vital morphological differences between kind I as well as type II SGNs along with their specific estimate patterns to the IHC or external hair cells OHC.

Without a doubt, the kind I, as well as II SGNs, were revealed to be molecularly various. The kind I SGNs reveals the semaphorin receptor Nrp2 and its co-receptor PlexinA3.

Upon binding Sema3F, secreted by the OHC, kind I SGNs are repelled and also limit their projections to the IHC. More just recently, making use of single sequencing has permitted a more detailed characterization of SGNs.

In this research study, I recognized that type I SGNs can be more identified right into three different subtypes. This information recommends a growing complexity of the acoustic system development and also assimilation of outside signals.

These instances highlight the intricacy of PNS growth. Intending to understand the surrounding atmosphere, each of these systems seems to have its very own advice devices, which via a limited and also coordinated regulation, establish a crucial pathway between sensory neurons and superior brain areas.

Unique genetic and also technological approaches also highlight the cellular diversification in these systems, most of them taken into consideration quite uniform until just recently.

The understanding of the molecular differences between cell enters a figured out structure is a crucial element in establishing therapeutic approaches such as stem cell therapy.

Also, these molecular differences can additionally assist in comprehending the possible results of various recognized support systems.

Finally, several groups have tried to understand the function of a spontaneous task in these frameworks.

The neural job has been observed to happen arbitrarily in many contexts, considering that early growth. This neuronal activity could be necessary to pattern and also enhance synapses, as was received the visual system.

Non-traditional functions of axon assistance particles

Axon support particles have been thoroughly examined throughout axonal development but have additionally been shown to be crucial in several varied organic processes such as angiogenesis as well as cell migration.

Undeniably, cortical growth depends on cellular migration. An essential concern for the past years has been the development of the neocortex, a specific feature of the animal brain.

Cortical advancement starts with the department of radial glial progenitor cells (RGPCs), which triggers all cortical neurons and glia. RGPCs are lined up at the cortical ventricular zone and also go through mitosis to either self-renew (symmetric division = indirect neurogenesis), or separate into cortical nerve cells (asymmetric division = direct neurogenesis).

Nonetheless, in animals, RGPCs can also divide symmetrically to trigger an intermediate progenitor cell (IPCs). IPCs can either self restore or separate into cortical nerve cells. Hence, IPCs have been recommended to work as the primary factor for cortex development in mammals.

Lately, they have determined a unique duty for Robo 1/2 in regulating radial glia cortical migration. By contrasting the computer mouse olfactory bulb (OB) (evocative, the reptilian paleocortex) to the cortex (Cx), observed that the OB only developed by direct neurogenesis whereas the Cx was developed primarily by indirect neurogenesis. Surprisingly, Robo1/2 was expressed in a slope, with a high-low expression in the OB compared to the Cx. Moreover, it was revealed that Robo1/2 could manage the notch approved signaling pathway through Delta-like 1 in addition to the ligands jagged 1 (Jag1) and also Jag2.

The device advanced is that high Robo1/2 expression in the OB minimizes Delta-like 1 expression and also raises Jag1 as well as Jag2 expression, causing asymmetric department and also straight neurogenesis.

Indeed, the gain of function experiments revealed that high Robo1/2 expression suffices to generate direct neurogenesis in the mouse Cx.

Interestingly, amniotes robbed of a neocortex, such as birds and reptiles, show high Robo1/2 expression in the cortex. Hence, the writers recommend the silencing of Robo1/2 as an evolutionary switch triggering indirect neurogenesis in creatures.

The Fibronectin Leucine Rich-repeat Transmembrane (FLRTs) proteins have likewise been identified as axon advice molecules. For example, thalamocortical axons sharing Dcc are not conscious of the netrin-1 slope present in the thalamus as a result of Robo1 silencing.

Nonetheless, FLRT3 can sequester Robo1 to allow for Dcc expression at the surface of thalamocortical neurons, thus activating netrin-1 responsiveness.

More recently, FLRTs have additionally been linked with cortical progenitor movement. In animals, the cortex initially develops as a laminar sheet. While some mammals (mice as well as rats) will preserve this smooth cortical growth, various other mammals (primates as well as ferrets) establish cortical folds up.

FLRT1/3 has lately been shown to be critical gamers in this procedure. Surprisingly, genetic ablation in computer mice of FLRT1/3 promotes cortical folding.

While the spreading rate of radial glia cells was the same, their migratory patterns were dramatically alarmed. Indeed, loss of FLRT1/3 raised neuronal clustering and also radial migration rate.

The developing columns of moving progenitors, causing an asymmetric spreading throughout the surface area of the cortex and, as a result developing sulci.

Of note, FLRT1/3 expression is reduced in gyrencephalic varieties, recommending that the abundance of FLRT1/3 during advancement advertised cortical smoothing (lissencephaly).

Techniques on just how to discover faster as well as better

1. Claim out loud what you want to keep in mind.
The study reveals that compared to reviewing or believing quietly (as if there are one more means to assume), the act of speech is a "fairly effective system for enhancing memory for chosen info."
According to the researcher, "Learning as well as memory benefit from energetic involvement. When we include an energetic procedure or a manufacturing element to a word, that word becomes much more distinctive in long-lasting memory, and also hence more unforgettable."
In short, while mentally rehearsing is good, practicing aloud is also better.
2. Bear in mind by hand, not on a computer system
Most of us can kind quicker than we can compose. (As well as a lot much more neatly).
However, study shows, handwriting your notes indicate you'll discover more Oddly enough, making note by hand improves both understandings as well as retention, perhaps since as opposed to just working as a quasi-stenographer, you're compelled to place points in your very own words to keep up.
Which means you'll remember what you listened to a lot longer.
Possibly that's why Richard Branson has maintained a long-lasting behavior of keeping a handwritten journal?
3. Chunk your research sessions
You're busy. So you wait till the eleventh hour to discover what you need to know: A discussion, a sales demonstration, a capitalist pitch.
Poor suggestion. Research study reveals "dispersed technique" is a much more efficient method to discover — the picture you want to toenail your capitalist pitch.
 Once you've drafted your pitch, gone through it once, then take a couple of minutes to make corrections as well as revisions.
Then move away for a couple of hours, or perhaps for a day, before you repeat the procedure.

Why does a distributed technique job? The "study-phase access the-ory" states that each time you attempt to obtain something from memory and the retrieval is extra sufficient, that memory becomes tougher to fail to remember.

 (If you review your pitch continuously, much of your discussion is still leading of mind.which means you don't need to obtain it from memory).

One more concept regards "contextual variability." When info obtains inscribed into memory, some of the contexts are additionally encoded.

 (Which is why paying attention to an old track can trigger you to re-member where you were, what you were feeling, and so on, when you first listened to that track.) That context develops valuable signs for re-trieving information.

No matter just how it functions, a distributed practice most definitely features. So give on your own adequate time to room out your discov-ering sessions. You'll find out more effectively and better.

4. Examination on your own a great deal

Several research studies reveal that self-testing is an incredibly effec-tive way to quicken the learning procedure.

Partially that results from the additional context produced; if you ex-amine yourself and also respond to improperly, not only are you more probable to remember the appropriate answer after you look it up.

you'll additionally bear in mind that you didn't keep in mind. (Getting glitch is a fantastic method to bear in mind it the next time, specifically if you have a tendency to be difficult on yourself.).

So do not just practice your presentation. Test yourself on what follows your intro. Examine yourself by noting the five bottom lines you wish to make.

 Attempt to recite vital stats, or sales estimates, or cash flow forecasts. Not just will you get confidence in how much you do recognize, you'll more quickly discover the things you do not remember.

Yet.

5. Modification of the method you exercise

Duplicating anything over and over once again in the hopes you will grasp that job will not just maintain you from boosting as rapidly as you could; in some cases, it may reduce your ability.

According to a recent research study from Johns Hopkins, if you practice a slightly customized variation of a job you intend to master, "you find out more as well as faster than if you keep exercising the specific very same point multiple times in a row.

" One of the most likely reasons is reconsolidation, a procedure where existing memories are recalled and also changed with brand-new knowledge.

State you want to master a new presentation. Do this:

1. Practice the standard skill.

Run through your discussion several times under the same problems you'll ultimately face when you do it live. Naturally, the 2nd time with will undoubtedly be better than the very first; that's precisely how the technique works. Yet after that, as opposed to experiencing it a third time.

2. Wait. Provide on your own at the very least six hrs so your memory can combine. (Which probably implies waiting up until tomorrow before you practice again, which is merely okay.).

3. Technique once again, yet this moment.

- Go a little faster. Speak a little-- only a few-- more swiftly than you typically do. Run through your slides somewhat quicker. Raising your speed suggests you'll make more mistakes, but that's OK-- at the same time, you'll customize old understanding with new knowledge-- and also lay the groundwork for improvement. Or.

- Go a little slower. The same point will undoubtedly occur. (And also, you can experiment with brand-new strategies-- including making use of silence for impact-- that aren't apparent when you provide at your regular rate.) Or.

- Break your discussion right into smaller portions. Nearly every job consists of a series of distinct steps. That's real for reviews. Select one section of your study. Deconstruct it. Master it. Then put the entire discussion back together. Or.

- Adjustment of the conditions. Make use of various projectors. Or multiple remotes. Or a lavaliere instead of a headset mic. Switch over the problems slightly; not just will that help you modify an existing memory, it will also make you better gotten ready for the unforeseen.

4. And maintain customizing the problems.

You can extend the procedure to almost anything. While it's efficient for finding out motor skills, the process can likewise be applied to discovering virtually anything.

6. Exercise regularly

This research shows that routine workout can improve memory recall. An additional study from McMaster College found that periods of high-intensity activity benefit physical fitness and memory: Workout led to considerable enhancements in a high-interference mind.

(Interference occurs when details that are comparable hinders of the features you're attempting to recall).

A commonly made use of instance for high-interference memory is re-membering faces, a skill that is especially helpful for individuals wishing to create links.

Workout also led to an increase in a chemical called BDNF (brain-derived neurotrophic element), a healthy protein that supports the feature, growth, and survival of brain cells.

So: Not just will you feel better if you exercise, you'll also boost your memory.

Win-win.

7. Obtain much more rest

Sleep is when the majority of the memory consolidation procedure occurs. That's why also a brief nap can enhance your memory recall.

In one study, participants memorized detailed cards to check their memory strength. After learning a collection of cards, they took a 40-minute break as well as one team slept while the other group remained awake.

After the break, both groups were checked on their memory of the cards. The sleep group executed dramatically much better, keeping typically 85 percent of the patterns contrasted to 60 percent for those who had actually stayed awake.

Researchers have also located that sleep deprivation can affect your capacity to devote new info to memory and combine any short-term memories you have made.

Profits? Sleep extra, learn more.

8. Learn numerous subjects one by one

As opposed to blocking (concentrating on one subject, one job, or one ability during an understanding session) find out or exercise several topics or skills in succession.

The procedure is called interleaving: Studying relevant concepts or abilities in parallel. And it turns out interleaving is a lot more reliable means to educate your brain (as well as your electric motor abilities). Why? One theory is that interleaving improves your brain's capability to separate in between ideas or skills. When you obstruct practice one skill, you can drill down until muscle memory takes over, and also, the ability becomes more or less automatic.

When you interleave several skills, anyone skill can't end up being meaningless-- and that's a good idea. Instead, you're continuously required to adjust and also change.

 You're frequently required to see, really feel, and also discriminate between different activities or various principles. Which aids you learn what you're attempting to gain because it assists you in obtaining understanding at a much deeper level.

9. Educate another person

It might sometimes be true that those who can not show .however, the study shows it's most definitely true that those who instruct speed up their understanding as well as preserve more.

Even just thinking that you'll need to educate someone can make you learn more appropriately. According to the researchers, "When teachers prepare to teach, they tend to seek bottom lines and also arrange info into a meaningful structure.

Our results recommend that students additionally count on these kinds of effective knowing techniques when they expect to instruct.".

The act of training also assists enhance expertise. Ask any person who has trained somebody else whether they additionally benefited from the experience.

They did.

10. Improve things you do understand

Connecting something brand-new to something you're familiar with is called associative knowing. Not the Pavlov's canine form of associative knowing, but the kind where you find out the relationship in between seemingly unrelated points.

In basic terms, whenever you claim, "Oh, I get it ... this is essentially like that," you're making use of associative learning.

11. Consume Alcohol Much Less Alcohol

Taking in way too many alcoholic beverages can be damaging to your health in numerous methods as well as can negatively affect your memory.

Binge alcohol consumption is a pattern of alcohol consumption that increases your blood alcohol levels to 0.08 grams per ml or above. Research studies have revealed it changes the mind and leads to memory shortages.

A research of 155 first-year university students located that pupils who ate six or even more drinks within a brief period, either weekly or regular monthly, had problems in an instant and delayed memory-recall tests compared to students who never binge drank.

Alcohol shows neurotoxic impacts on the brain. Repetitive episodes of binge alcohol consumption can damage the hippocampus, a part of the brain that plays an essential duty in memory.

While having a drink or two once in a while is perfectly healthy, avoiding excessive alcohol consumption is a wise method to protect your memory.

Alcohol has neurotoxic effects on the brain, consisting of decreasing memory efficiency. Occasional modest drinking isn't a problem, yet binge drinking can harm your hippocampus, a crucial area of your brain related to memory.

Are you required to find out something brand-new? Attempt to connect it, a minimum of partially, with something you already recognize. After that, you only need to discover the differences or subtleties. And you'll have the ability to use better context-- which will undoubtedly assist with memory storage space and also retrieval-- to the brand-new info you discover.

Every one of which implies you'll require to discover a great deal much less.

Which science states will undoubtedly cause you to have the ability to learn a lot more quickly.

12. Maintain a Healthy Weight
Keeping a healthy body weight. Is essential for wellness and also is one of the best ways to keep your mind and body in leading problem.
Numerous studies have established weight problems as a risk variable for a cognitive decrease.
Remarkably, being obese can trigger changes to memory-associated genes in mind, adversely affecting memory.
Obesity can additionally bring about insulin resistance as well as inflammation, both of which can adversely influence the mind.
A study of 50 people starting from ages of 18 as well as 35 discovered that a higher body mass index was associated with considerably even worse efficiency on memory examinations.
Weight problems are likewise connected with a more significant threat of developing Alzheimer's illness, a current condition that destroys memory and also cognitive feature.
Weight problems is a risk element for a cognitive decrease. Keeping a body mass index within the usual array may aid you to stay clear of a host of the issues associated with excessive weight, consisting of imperfect memory.

13. Try a Fish Oil Supplement
Fish oil is rich in the omega-3 fats eicosapentaenoic acid (EPA) and also docosahexaenoic acid (DHA).
These fats are essential for total health and also have been revealed to reduce the threat of heart disease, minimize swelling, ease stress and anxiety and anxiety, and even slow-moving psychological decline.
Lots of researches have shown that eating fish and also fish oil supplements may boost memory, particularly in older people.
One study of 36 older adults with moderate cognitive problems discovered that short-term, as well as working memory ratings, improved dramatically after they took concentrated fish oil supplements for a year.
Another current testimonial of 28 research studies revealed that when grownups with mild signs of memory loss took supplements abundant in DHA and also EPA, like fish oil, they experienced enhanced episodic memory.

Both DHA and EPA are vital to the health as well as the functioning of the brain as well as also help in reducing inflammation in the body, which has been linked to cognitive decline.

Fish and fish oil supplements are abundant in the omega-3 fatty acids EPA and also DHA. Consuming them might help boost short-term, functioning, and anecdotal memory, specifically in older people.

14. Consume Less Sugarcoated

Consuming excessively sugarcoated has been connected to many health problems and persistent conditions, including cognitive decline. Research study has revealed that a sugar-laden diet plan can bring about poor memory and also decreased mind quantity, especially in the area of the mind that shops temporary memory.

For instance, one study of greater than 4,000 individuals found that those with higher consumption of sugary drinks like soft drinks had lower total brain quantities as well as more miserable memories usually contrasted to individuals who consumed much less sugar.

Cutting down on sugar not just assists your memory but also enhances your general health.

Research study has shown that people that regularly eat great deals of added sugar may have more miserable memories as well as reduced brain quantities than those who eat less sugar.

15. Exercise Mindfulness

Mindfulness is a mental state in which you focus on your existing scenario, preserving recognition of your environments as well as sensations.

Mindfulness is utilized in meditation, but the two aren't the same. Reflection is a more formal method, whereas mindfulness is a psychological habit you can use in any scenario.

Research studies have shown that mindfulness works at decreasing stress and boosting concentration as well as memory.

One research of 293 psychology pupils revealed that those that went through mindfulness training had boosted recognition-memory performance when recalling objects compared to trainees that did not get mindfulness training (Mindfulness has likewise been linked with a lower risk of age-related cognitive decline and total improvement in emotional wellness 20.

Include mindfulness techniques right into your everyday regimen by paying, even more, focus on your existing circumstance, concentrating on your breathing and gently resetting your attention when your mind wanders.

Exercising mindfulness techniques has been associated with boosted memory performance. Mindfulness is likewise linked to minimized age-related cognitive decrease.

16. Reduce Refined Carbs

Consuming vast amounts of polished carbs like cakes, cereal, cookies, white rice, and also white bread may be harming to your memory.

These foods have a high glycemic index, indicating the body absorbs these carbohydrates promptly, resulting in a spike in blood sugar degrees.

Researches have revealed that the Western diet regimen, which is high in polished carbs, is related to dementia, cognitive decrease, and also lowered cognitive function.

One research study of 317 healthy children found that those that consumed a lot more refined carbohydrates like white rice, noodles, and fast food had minimized cognitive capability, including more imperfect temporary and functioning memory.

Additional research demonstrated that adults who took in ready-to-eat morning meal cereal daily had more inferior cognitive function than those that ate grain less frequently.

Like sugarcoated, fine-tuned carbs lead to a spike in blood glucose degrees, which can harm your mind in time. Diet plans high in refined carbs have been associated with dementia, cognitive decline, and also minimized mind features.

17. Get Your Vitamin D Levels Tested

Vitamin D is an essential nutrient that plays lots of crucial functions in the body.

Low degrees of vitamin D has actually been linked to a host of wellness problems, including a decrease in the cognitive feature.

Research that complied with 318 older grownups for five years located that those who had blood levels of vitamin D less than 20 nanograms per ml shed their memory and also various other cognitive capabilities faster than those with typical vitamin D degrees.

Reduced degrees of vitamin D has additionally been connected to a better threat of creating mental deterioration.

Vitamin-D deficiency is usual, especially in colder environments and also in those with darker skin. Speak with your physician concerning obtaining a blood test to find out if you require a vitamin D supplement.

The vitamin-d shortage is widespread, especially in chillier environments, as well as has been related to age-related cognitive decline as well as mental deterioration. If you assume you might have reduced degrees of vitamin D, ask your physician for a blood test.

18. Think about Curcumin

Curcumin is a compound discovered in high focus in turmeric origin. It's one of a category of substances called polyphenols.

It is a powerful anti-oxidant and also puts in powerful anti-inflammatory results in the body.

Numerous animal researches have discovered that curcumin lowers oxidative damages and also inflammation in the brain and additionally decreases the number of amyloid plaques. These build upon neurons as well as create cell and cell fatality, resulting in amnesia.

Amyloid plaque buildup may contribute to the development of Alzheimer's condition.

Though more human research studies are needed on the impacts of curcumin on memory, animal research studies suggest it may be effective at increasing consciousness and also protecting against cognitive decline.

Curcumin is a powerful antioxidant. Animal researches have shown it lowers swelling as well as amyloid plaques in the brain. Nonetheless, more study on human beings is needed.

19. Include Some Cocoa to Your Diet

Chocolate is not only delicious; however, likewise healthy, offering an effective dose of antioxidants called flavonoids. The study suggests flavonoids are especially beneficial to the mind.

They may assist in stimulating the development of blood vessels and also nerve cells as well as boost blood flow part of the brain involved with memory.

A research of 30 healthy individuals discovered that those who took in dark chocolate has 720 mg of chocolate flavonoids showed better memory contrasted to those who ate delicious white chocolate without cocoa flavonoids.

To obtain one of the essential benefits out of chocolate, select dark delicious chocolate with a chocolate content of 70% cacao or higher. That will undoubtedly guarantee to assist it includes larger quantities of antioxidants like flavonoids.

Cocoa is high in anti-oxidants that might aid enhance memory efficiency. See to it to choose delicious dark chocolate with 70% cacao or higher, so you get a focused dosage of anti-oxidants.

How to maintain psychological flexibility

Cognitive versatility refers to our ability to disengage from one task as well as respond to an additional or think about various concepts at the exact time.

Someone who is cognitively adjustable will be able to find out more swiftly, resolve issues extra artistically, as well as adjust and also reply to brand-new circumstances better, which is why it's so important in both educational settings and also the workplace.

According to a 2016 record from the Globe Economic Forum that looked at the future of work across nine different markets in 15 of the globe's most substantial economic situations, employers will certainly quickly be positioning more focus on cognitive abilities like creative thinking and versatility.

So whether you're a trainee or working expert, building your cognitive adaptability is an excellent method to create professional as well as stay up to date with the ever-altering work environment of the future.

One of the very best practices to end up being much more cognitively flexible is to expose yourself to new experiences and ways of doing points, yet if you're not exactly sure where to start, here are a few ideas.

1. Change your everyday routine

If you're looking for an easy way to begin developing your cognitive flexibility, you can start by altering your routine and also doing ordinary things diversly.

For instance, if you're habituated to taking the exact course to work each day, seek a different path or take into consideration making the bus rather than driving yourself.

If you generally obtain your workout at the fitness center, modify things up by running in the park or choosing a bike ride.

Even making the smallest of modifications like resting at a new place at the dinner table or using your left hand to comb your teeth as opposed to your right can assist you in building as well as strengthen new neural pathways.

2. Seek out brand-new encounter

Each time you undergo something out of the ordinary or discover something brand-new, the brain produces new synaptic connections. Unique and exciting experiences have also been revealed to trigger the launch of dopamine, which not just enhances inspiration but likewise boosts memory and even understanding.

So going out of your way to undergo new points or take part in novel activities can go a long way towards aiding you to create cognitive adaptability.

These could indicate traveling to one more country or offering in a new industry; however, it could likewise take the kind of tasks like learning a new language or musical instrument, taking a dancing course, or per-haps exploring a part of town you're not acquainted with.

3. Practice thinking creatively

Another means to construct cognitive flexibility is to make an effort to think in unusual and also imaginative means or practice different rea-soning.

One research study by psychologist Dr. Robert Steinberg showed that when trainees were taught to assume in both innovative and also prac-tical methods, not just did their grades boost, but they were additionally able to move the understanding they gained to entirely different areas of agreement.

Different thinking usually happens in a spontaneous and also free-flowing manner and also entails reasoning in regards to unlimited possibilities as opposed to a limited set of choices. Wish to know even more? Take a look at this article for suggestions on exactly how to influence divergent thinking.

4. Don't always take the straightforward means

Nowadays, we have technology as well as apps that make our lives much easier in numerous methods, from spell check and also autocorrect to GPS. Yet the fact is that making things easier for ourselves isn't always the most useful thing for our cognitive versatility.

Research reveals that presenting supposed "preferable problems" can bring about much more profound understanding, so by making a point of not always choosing the most comfortable means of doing points, you can keep your mind sharp as well as even learn through your daily experiences.

For example, if you're driving to an area you're not familiar with, try to navigate your means making use of a map as well as requesting for instructions instead of using your GPS, or instead of reaching for your phone the min you need to make a calculation, get a pen and paper, and also do it the old-fashioned method.

5. Go out of your process to fulfill brand-new individuals

Satisfying people from various societies as well as walks of life whose perspectives and also point of view are most likely to differ from your own can aid you to be less rigid in your mind-set and also approve that there might be more than one "right" way of looking at things.

Research shows that individuals who are exposed to circumstances that challenge their concepts concerning what's right and incorrect often tend to have higher cognitive adaptability. One study specifically found that college students that had been subjected to variety, as well as social differences, were most likely to have gotten to a sophisticated phase of ethical reasoning.

So make an effort to meet people beyond your usual social circles, whether that means taking a trip abroad, offering, training, or connecting with people through social media sites.

6. Transfer your knowing

Finding out to transfer what you have found out in one context into a brand-new context can be an excellent exercise in cognitive adaptability since it requires you to create brand-new connections between formerly unconnected networks of expertise and assume more artistically. Without the ability to move abilities and understanding to new contexts, your discovering will not have as significant an effect.

For example, one research study found that although street children could do complicated mathematical computations when marketing their products, they weren't able to address some issues that were presented to them in a college context.

If you wish to establish your capability to transfer understanding, research shows that discussing a brand-new idea in your own words not only aids you recognize any inaccurate assumptions, however likewise assists you to generalize a plan for future application.

Once you make sure you realize the concept, you can look for methods to apply it in real-world situations.

7. Obstacle your precepts

Study shows that seeking experiences that examine your morals and reveal you to a range of beliefs, worths, and also assumptions can give you a better understanding of culturally different viewpoints as well as aid you end up being extra flexible in your reasoning.

Even if you don't always agree with a person's perspective or belief system, being cognitively adaptable ways you'll have the ability to think of why they could see points in this way and comprehend their viewpoint. This capacity will make it much easier for you to communicate with people, resolve conflicts, and also adapt your thinking to various circumstances.

Naturally, travel is one means to test your point of view, yet even just checking out moral problems as well as thinking about them can assist you to create in this area.

Just remember that the extra you head out of your means do things differently, take part in new experiences, as well as interact with different people, the much more versatile your reasoning will end up being.

How to make the brain concentrate

You'll never obtain large muscular tissues from remaining on the sofa all the time, as well as you'll never create incredible powers of concentration from individually checking out Buzzfeed and seeing Tosh.O. Your mind muscular tissues, similar to your physical muscle mass, need resistance; they need difficulties that stretch their limitations and also in so doing, expand their emphasis fibers.

Below we outline exercises that will boost your focus to ensure that you can begin lifting more significant and even much heavier cognitive loads.

1.Enhance the stamina of your emphasis progressively

If you choose you to wish to get in shape; however, are beginning at ground zero, the worst point you can do is to throw yourself right into a severe training program-- you'll wind up wounded, inhibited, or both, as well as you'll give up before you even really get started.

Furthermore, if your attention span is currently somewhat slack, it's best to develop the weight you ask it to lift gradually. In this series, we've pointed out trying the "Pomodoro Method" in which you work for, claim, 45 minutes straight, and afterward enable yourself a 15-minute break. But for a number of us, 45 minutes could also be a mind marathon!

To begin with a quite straightforward objective and function your method up from there. Establish a timer for 5 mins and emphasis entirely on your work/reading for that period. After that, take a 2-minute break before going at it once more for one more 5 minutes.

Daily, add one more 5 minutes to your concentrated job time, in addition to an added 2 mins to your break time. In 9 days, you must be able to help 45 minutes straight prior to you allow yourself an 18-minute break.

Once you get comfortable with that set up, you can function to extend your focus sessions a little, while reducing your break times.

2. Develop a distraction order of business
Since the net has made any little bit of details instantaneously available, we tend to wish to look something up the moment it crosses our mind.
 "I question what the weather condition will be like tomorrow?" "What year did that movie appeared?" "I wonder what's new in some medial social feed?" As a result, we'll toggle away from what we're working with the immediate inquiries or ideas pop into our minds. The issue is, as soon as we get sidetracked, it handles typical 25(!) minutes to go back to our first job. And also, changing our focus too and fro drains its toughness.
So to remain on task, whenever something you wish to look into stands out into your head, write it down on a piece of paper next to you (or possibly in Evernote for you technology types), as well as promise on your own you'll have the ability to look it up as soon as your concentrating session is over as well as your break time has shown up.
3. Build your willpower
 Voluntary interest, as well as willpower, are thoroughly laced. Our willpower enables us to purposely neglect interruptions while remaining concentrated on the job at hand. It would offer your interest span well to evaluate our long post on strengthening your self-discipline.
4. Meditate
 Not only does meditation aid maintain you amazing, calm, and accumulated, the study has additionally shown repeatedly that mindfulness meditation can improve your interest span substantially.
In one research study, 140 volunteers took part in an eight-week course in reflection training. After the week, all the volunteers showed quantifiable enhancements in attention span, in addition to various other executive psychological functions.
You do not have to spend your days practicing meditation in a monastery to take advantage of its attention-boosting power. The study has revealed that just 10 to 20 minutes of reflection a day will suffice.
What's even more, you'll also see renovations in your focus after only four days.
So if you desire the power to focus on your studies for hrs at a time, begin your mornings off just concentrating on your breath for a few minutes.

5. Practice mindfulness throughout the day
 Along with dedicating 10 to 20 minutes a day to mindfulness meditation, interest specialists recommend finding chances to practice mindfulness throughout your day.
Mindfulness is just focusing entirely on what you're doing, slowing down, and observing every one of the physical as well as emotional feelings you are experiencing because minute.
You can practice attention when you eat as you take some time to chew your food indeed and also focus on its tastes as well as structure.
 You can practice consciousness when you shave; as you smell your shaving cream, keep in mind the enjoyment of applying a cozy soap to your face, and gradually drag the razor throughout your bristle.
Integrating brief sessions of mindfulness throughout your day will certainly enhance as well as increase your focus period for the times when you require it.
Mindfulness can likewise assist you in pushing back versus interruptions as they emerge. If you're dealing with a task as well as feel that agitated impulse to go do another thing, think to yourself, "Be here currently." Because moment, bring your awareness to your body as well as your breath. After a couple of secs of concentrating on your breathing, you'll see that the interruption is no more existing and that you're ready to return to function.

6. Exercise (your body)
 Not only can you contrast exercising your mind to using your body, doing the latter straight benefits the previous.
Researchers have discovered that students who participated in moderate exercise before taking a test that gauged focus periods carried out much better than students that didn't workout.
The scientists found that exercise mostly aids our brain's ability to neglect interruptions, although they aren't precisely sure why.
 I would indeed venture to say that the self-control it requires to push via the pain of an exercise strengthens the same supply of determination that we use to overlook the itch of interruptions to maintain working/focusing.
7. Remember stuff

We have spoken about memorization on the website previously. Besides being an excellent bar method and also giving you a fount of poems to state at the drop of a hat, remembering stuff is a unique method to exercise your mind muscular tissues. Make it a goal to memorize a verse or a poem of bible weekly.

8. Strategy and Imagine a Couple Of Essential Jobs Every Day

Our ideas shape our reality. Why? Because our thoughts generate feelings, feelings bring about activity, and also action causes results. As a part of your early morning regimen, establish one to 3 critical tasks that should be done throughout the day. Do not merely think about them ostensibly.

Picture them and replicate the sensations you'll get after ending up each job. If you consider your day's success, your subconscious will do everything it can to aid you in turning thoughts into truth.

What Regarding Focus Training Gaming?

Mind training video games have received a lot of press in current years. You've in all probability seen commercials for Lumosity or Brain Age on Nintendo DS.

The video games' designers declare that investing merely a couple of minutes a day playing can enhance your attention, memory, as well as imagination. Nevertheless, the study on the honesty of these claims is divided.

Some studies indicate that mind training games can assist in enhancing focus in kids with ADHD or in the senior, but that they don't benefit young, healthy adults.

Various other researches reveal that while particular brain-training video games can improve focus degrees, those gains do not crossover to different other areas of life. To put it in the mind training video games can aid people to pay far better attention and also do better at brain training games, but they will not help individuals pay much better focus in class or while researching.

Recent research showed a specific type of mind training game called n-back could improve functioning memory (a crucial aspect of attention), which enhancement can crossover to other cognitive difficulties.

So what does this all mean? The decision is still out on whether these mind games will definitively raise attention periods, and additional research studies needed to be done.

It won't hurt to try them out as part of your attention training program, yet include the other suggestions detailed below as well.

9. Read long stuff slowly

 Combat the TL; DR society. With the surge of tablets, e-readers, and also smart devices, some researches suggest that reading e-content as a whole has risen nearly 40%.

 This is an advantage. You 'd think so, except that Slate recently did some research study with the help of internet site analytics company Chartbeat that established that just a modest 5% of viewers who begin a short article online would complete them. What's more, 38% of readers never go beyond an initial couple of paragraphs.

 So to state that reading generally has increased would be deceptive. What we're doing is more scrolling, and also less engaging.

At the same time, we read fewer publications; a recent study revealed that 25% of Americans did not review solitary writing last year.

This is absolutely a shame. While long most definitely does not immediately equivalent much better, particular complex ideas are impossible to condense right into shortlist articles and also need an entire book (or several books) to expand.

To avoid something just since it is long is to lose out on a universe of knowledge readily available only to those going to dive deeper.

There's certainly a place for skimming online, and discovering a little regarding a great deal. However you should additionally make room for plunging into a couple of subjects whole hog.

If you have not reviewed a publication in some time, I test you to select one up tonight. Attempt to go into it. Find out exactly how to read a book properly; it'll change your life.

Besides publications, make an initiative to read a couple of lengthy posts a week. Longform journalism, as it's called, is occurrence a renaissance of types, and the quantity of top quality, thorough material readily available is at an all-time high.

The Art of Manliness (Constantly strives to publish detailed posts that are as valuable as feasible. Also, I hear its founder has a beautiful mustache.).

10. Keep interested

The more baffled you are about the world, the higher the stamina of your concentration will certainly be when it comes to any endeavor. William James suggests a simple experiment to evaluate how staying curious about the item of your attention can lengthen your capability to remain focused on it:

" Try to go to steadfastly to a dot on the paper or the wall. You presently find that a person or the other of two points has happened: either your field of vision has ended up been blurred.

To ensure that you currently see nothing distinctive in any way; otherwise, you have unwillingly ceased to take a look at the dot concerned, as well as are taking a look at something else.

But, if you ask on your succeeding questions regarding the dot,-- how big it is, how far, of what shape, what shade of shade, and so on; to put it simply, if you transform it over, if you consider it in various methods, as well as in addition to various kinds of associates,-- you can maintain your mind on it for a relatively long time.

This is what the wizard does, in whose hands an offered subject coruscates and grows.".

Charles Darwin was a master of this principle. His contemporaries admired his ability to spend a whole day just looking at animals and also plants.

Darwin's secret was his constant inquisitiveness-- he might discover an increasing number of about a single item by homing know different details, examining it in various methods, asking new concerns. Gradually he would peel back its layers.

11. Practice mindful listening

Emphasis isn't just useful for intellectual endeavors. It's also an essential interpersonal skill. The capacity to be existing with a liked one or pal constructs your relationship, intimacy, and also depend on and even with them.

At the same time, making an effort to concentrate all your energy on someone else enhances your concentration muscles generally. It's a win-win.

So next time you're chatting with your main squeeze, do away with your phone as well as pay attention as attentively as possible.

12. Carry out concentration exercises

The above exercises not only improve your emphasis, yet offer other benefits as well. Now and then, nevertheless, it's good to do some activities that are intended purely at enhancing your focus. Right here are twelve to try.

13. Locate Your Peak Hours

Some people carry out far better throughout the day, while others do lovely during the evening. To locate your most efficient hours-- the "peak hrs"-- you need to measure your efficiency during numerous hours of the day proactively.

Take note of your energy, believed patterns, interruptions, inspiration, and state of mind while experimenting with various work hrs. Make sure you allow at least a week to develop these peak hours.

So, if you attempt to obtain your essential jobs done from 8 AM to 10 AM, experiment it for a week. Following week, concentrate your attention on vital tasks beginning with 10 AM as well as finishing at noon.

14. Avoid Multitasking

Multitasking has been verified to minimize our cognitive capacities due to the reality that the brain can concentrate on one task each time.

Although multitasking can be useful in various scenarios, you need to prevent it as high as you can whenever you deal with vital tasks.

Provide your complete interest to the task at hand to enhance the high quality and also rate of work!

15. Acknowledge Your Need to Prevent Discomfort as well as to Gain Pleasure

When we do something, we do it since we seek pleasure or since we wish to stay clear of pain.

Think about it-- when students have to do their homework, they hesitate since their subconscious minds signal inbound distress. When the deadline is close, they'll take action to avoid the pain of receiving a negative quality.

Take this example as well as synchronize it with your life. Each time you wish to focus on a job, acknowledge your immediate reaction.

Are you attempting to stay clear of pain? Or you're searching for satisfaction? When you end up being the viewer, you'll be able to supervise.

16. Train your brain

Playing particular types of games can help you improve at concentrating. Try:
- sudoku.
- crossword problems.
- chess.
- jigsaw puzzles.
- word searches or shuffles.
- memory games.

Results of a 2015 study trusted Resource of 4,715 grownups recommend spending 15 mins a day, five days a week, on mind training tasks can have a significant effect on concentration.

Mind training games can likewise help you create your working and short-term memory, as well as your processing as well as analytical abilities.

Kids

Mind training can help kids, also. Buy a publication of word challenges, complete a jigsaw problem together, or play a game of memory.

Also, coloring can help improve focus on youngsters or adults. Older children may delight in extra in-depth coloring web pages, like those discovered in adult coloring publications.

Older grownups.

The effects of mind training games may be especially vital for older adults since memory, as well as focus, often tend to decline with age. Research study from2014Trusted Source that considered 2,832 older grownups acted on individuals after ten years. Older adults who completed in between 10 and 14 sessions of cognitive training saw enhanced cognition, memory, as well as processing skills.

After ten years, most of the research study participants reported they could finish daily tasks a minimum of as well as they might at the beginning of the test, if not much better.

17. Get your game on

Mind video games might not be the only kind of video game that can assist enhance concentration. The newer research study likewise suggests playing computer games might aid improve focus.

A 2018 research checking out 29 people located evidence to suggest an hr of pc gaming might help boost selective aesthetic focus (VSA). VSA refers to your capability to focus on a specific job while overlooking distractions around you.

Its small size limited this research study, so these findings aren't conclusive. The research additionally really did not determine for how long this increase in VSA lasted.

Research authors advise future studies to proceed to check out how computer games can help boost mental activity as well as increase focus.

A 2017 review trusted Source looked at 100 studies checking out the effects computer game might have on cognitive function.

The results of the evaluation suggest playing a computer game may lead to different changes in the brain, consisting of raised attention as well as focus.

This review had several restrictions, consisting of the truth that the research studies focused on extensively varying topics, consisting of computer game dependency as well as likely results of violent video games. Researches specifically created to explore the benefits of a computer game can aid in supporting these findings.

18. Boost rest

Rest deprival can quickly disrupt concentration, in addition to other cognitive functions, such as memory and interest.

Periodic sleep starvation may not create way too many problems for you. However, consistently failing to get a good night's rest can affect your state of mind as well as efficiency at the office.

Being also tired can also reduce your reflexes and even impact your capability to drive or do other day-to-day tasks.

A demanding timetable, health, and wellness issues, and also other factors occasionally make it hard to get sufficient rest. However, it's essential to try as well as obtain as near the advised amount as possible on a lot of evenings.

Numerous professionals recommend adults aim for 7 to 8 hours of sleep each night.

Improving the rest, you do obtain can also have an advantage. A few quick tips:

- Switch off the TV and even put away displays an hour before bed.

- Maintain your space at a comfy, however trendy temperature level.
- Wind down before bed with soft music, a warm bath, or a publication.
- Go to sleep as well as stand up around the very same time every day, even on weekends.
- Workout frequently, however, try to avoid a hefty exercise right before bed.

19. Hang around in nature

If you wish to improve your focus naturally, attempt to obtain outdoors daily, even for just 15 to 20 minutes. You may take a short go through a park.

 Sitting in your garden or yard can also assist. Any natural environment has advantages.

Scientific evidence significantly supports the positive influence of native environments.

Research Study from 2014Trusted Resource found proof to suggest consisting of plants in the workplace helped increase concentration and productivity, along with workplace fulfillment as well as air top quality.

Try including a plant or 2 to your work area or house for a variety of positive benefits. Succulents make excellent choices for low-maintenance plants if you don't have a green thumb.

Youngsters.

Kids take advantage of natural environments, also. A research study released in 2017 followed over 1,000 children from birth to age 7.

The research study intended to figure out exactly how long-lasting exposure to trees and also greenery at home or in your area may impact focus on children.

The research found evidence to recommend natural surroundings might benefit mind advancement as well as might likewise boost focus on youngsters.

Nature might have even more advantages for children with ADHD. A 2009 study trusted Resource that took a look at 17 children with ADHD discovered proof that a 20-minute walk in the park could help enhance concentration more significant than a trail of the same size in a city setting.

20. Listen to music

Activating songs while working or studying may help increase concentration.

Even if you don't delight in paying attention to music while you function, making use of nature noises or white noise to mask history seems can additionally improve concentration and also various other mental functions, according to study.

The sort of songs you listen to can make a difference. Experts generally concur symphonic music, notably baroque symphonic music or nature sounds, are excellent choices to aid your focus.

If you uncommitted for symphonic music, attempt ambient or digital music without lyrics, maintain the songs softly, or at history noise degree, so it does not wind up sidetracking you.

It's also crucial to stay clear of picking songs you enjoy or dislike, considering that both kinds can end up distracting you.

21. Vary your diet

The foods you eat can impact cognitive features like concentration and also memory. Avoiding refined grains, excessive sugar, and too very greasy or fatty foods. To enhance focus, attempt consuming even more of the following:

- oily fish (believe salmon and trout).
- eggs (white and also yolk both).
- blueberries.
- spinach.

You can locate more brain foods on this listing.

Remaining moistened can additionally have a favorable influence on focus. Even moderate dehydration can make it more challenging to focus or remember details.

Consuming breakfast can help by improving your focus first thing in the morning. Aim for a dish that's reduced in added sugars and high in protein as well as fiber. Oatmeal, ordinary yogurt with fruit, or whole-grain toast with eggs are all great breakfast options.

22. Drink high levels of caffeine

There's no need to consist of high levels of caffeine in your diet plan if you like to prevent it, but researchTrusted Resource does recommend high levels of caffeine that can profit your attention and also focus.

If you feel your focus beginning to drop, think about a cup of coffee or eco-friendly tea. A serving of dark chocolate-- 70 percent cacao or higher-- can have comparable benefits if you don't enjoy caffeinated beverages.

A2017 study trusted Resource discovered proof to recommend phyto-chemicals naturally found in matcha, a sort of eco-friendly tea, not only improve cognitive function however can help promote relaxation. So matcha may be a great option if the coffee tends to make you feel anxious or on edge.

23. Try supplements

Some supplements may assist promote much better concentration as well as boosted mind function.

You'll intend to talk to your healthcare provider before attempting any supplements, specifically if you have any health and wellness problems or allergic reactions.

A doctor can look at the possible advantages and threats of supplements with you and might advise one that's finest for your needs.

It's frequently possible to obtain all the vitamins you require by including specific foods to your diet plan, yet supplements can often assist you to meet day-to-day intake objectives.

The following supplements may assist promote raised focus and total brain health:

- folate.
- choline.
- vitamin K.
- flavonoids.
- omega-3 fats.
- guarana seed essence.

24. Do a concentration workout

Focus workouts often aid youngsters who have difficulty concentrating. This mental exercise involves completely dedicating attention to an activity for a set period.

Try these activities:

- Draw or scribble for 15 minutes.
- Spend a few mins throwing a balloon or small ball with one more person.
- Establish a timer for 3 to 5 minutes. Attempt to blink just feasible.

- Suck on a lollipop or hard candy till it's gone-- withstand the urge to attack into it. Take notice of the taste, the experience of the sweet on your tongue, and also for how long it requires to consume it.

After finishing one of the activities, ask your youngster to write a summary or sketch just how they felt throughout the experience. Young children can use words to describe their feelings.

Talking about where they shed focus as well as just how they took care of to redouble can help them develop these abilities for use in daily tasks.

A concentration workout can profit adults, as well, so do not hesitate to give it a try yourself.

Series Final thought

Modernity has provided us a lot of conveniences and also eases, yet it has additionally released a torrent of stimulations completing for our focus. To live a genuinely flourishing life amidst this cacophony of disturbances, grasping your attention is vital.

At the end of your life, that you have ended up being, what you have actually discovered and also achieved, and also who exists at the end with you will certainly be the sum total of what you picked to pay attention to every year, day, as well as hr of your life.

Will a series of pet cat video clips flash prior to your eyes? Or will you look back on the deep discussions you had with your family and friends, guides that changed your life, and the little information you found in all the places you visited?

We hope our collection on interest has obtained you to think about this progressively priceless asset in a brand-new light, as well as influenced you to take action to improve it. You'll be surprised how much your life can improve just by focusing on your interests.

What is Meditation as well as How It Influences Our Minds

What is meditation?
There are different methods to practice meditation, and considering that it's such a specific technique, there are probably more significant than any of us find out.
There are a pair that are typically focused on heavily in clinical research, though.
These are focused-attention, or conscious reflection, which is where you concentrate on one specific thing-- maybe your breathing, and experience in your body or particular things beyond you.
 The point of this type of meditation is to focus highly on one point and constantly bring your interest back to that focal point when it roams.
The other sort of meditation that's frequently used in research is open-monitoring meditation.
 This is where you take notice of every one of things happening around you-- you see every little something without responding.

What takes place in your mind when you practice meditation

This is where things get interesting. Utilizing contemporary innovation like fMRI scans, scientists have developed a much more comprehensive understanding of what's happening in our brains when we practice meditation, sort of comparable to how researchers have formerly considered determining imagination in our minds.

The total distinction is that our brains quit processing information as actively as they normally would. We start to reveal a decline in beta waves, which suggests that our minds are refining details, even after a single 20-minute reflection session if we have never tried it before.

In the picture listed below, you can see precisely how the beta waves (received brilliant shades on the left) are substantially decreased during reflection (on the right).

Below is the very best explanation I found of what takes place in each part of the brain during meditation:

Frontal lobe

This is the most highly developed part of the mind, in charge of thinking, planning, feelings, and also uneasy recognition. Throughout reflection, the frontal cortex tends to go offline.

Parietal lobe

This part of the brain refines sensory information about the surrounding world, orienting you in time and also the room. Throughout reflection, activity in the parietal lobe slows down.

Thalamus

The gatekeeper for the senses, this organ concentrates your interest by channeling some sensory information deeper right into the brain as well as quitting various other signals in their tracks. Reflection lowers the flow of inbound info to a drip.

Reticular formation

As the mind's sentry, this framework receives incoming stimulations as well as places the brain on alert, prepared to react. Meditating dials back the arousal signal.

Exactly how meditation affects us

Now that we know what's going on inside our brains, let's have a look at the research study right into the ways it impacts our health and wellness. It remains, in reality, really comparable to how exercising influences our minds.

Much better concentrate

Because reflection is a method in concentrating, It's a long-lasting effect our focus as well as knowing when it drifts, this improves our emphasis when we're not practicing meditation; also that originates from routine rounds of meditation.

Concentrated is very much like a muscle, one that needs to be reinforced via workout.

Less anxiety

This point is pretty technical; however, it's exciting. The more we practice meditation, the less anxiousness we have, and also, it ends up this is since we're loosening up the connections of absolute neural paths. This seems contrary; however, it's not.

What takes place without meditation is that there's a section of our brains that's in some cases called the Me Facility (it's technically the medial prefrontal cortex).

This is the component that refines details associating with ourselves and our experiences. Generally the neural pathways from the physical sensation as well as concern facilities of the mind to the Me Center are really strong.

When you experience a scary or disturbing experience, it sets off a strong reaction in your Me Center, making you feel terrified and under attack.

When we practice meditation, we deteriorate this neural connection. This implies that we don't react as strongly to experiences that may have once lit up our Me Centers.

As we deteriorate this connection, we all at once enhance the link in between what's referred to as our Evaluation Facility (the part of our minds understood for reasoning) as well as our physical feeling and also fear facilities.

So when we experience terrifying or distressing experiences, we can much more quickly look at them logically. Below's an example:
As an example, when you experience pain, as opposed to coming to be nervous and also thinking it implies something is wrong with you, you can view the pain fluctuate without becoming captured in a tale about what it might mean.
A lot more imagination
As a writer, this is one thing I'm always thinking about as well as we have discovered the scientific research of creativity in depth before, Sadly it's not the easiest thing to research; however, there is some study right into how reflection can affect our creative thinking.
 Researchers at the Netherlands University examined both focused-attention and also open-monitoring arbitration to see if there was any kind of enhancement in imagination later on.
 They located that people who practiced focused-attention reflection did not show any apparent indications of renovation in the creative thinking task following their meditation.
 For those that did open-monitoring meditation, nonetheless, they executed better on a job that asked to come up with originalities.
A lot more compassion
Research study on meditation has revealed that empathy and concern are higher in those who practice reflection routinely. One experiment showed individuals pictures of other people that were either great, negative, or neutral in what they called "concern reflection."
The participants were able to focus their focus and lower their emotional reactions to these photos, even when they weren't in a reflective state. They also experienced even more compassion for others when shown disturbing pictures.
Part of this originates from activity in the amygdala-- the part of the mind that refines psychological stimuli.
Throughout reflection, this part of the brain usually reveals reduced tasks, yet in this experiment, it was remarkably receptive when individuals were shown images of people.
One more research study in 2008 found that people who practiced meditation routinely had more powerful activation levels in their temporal, parietal junctures (a part of the brain linked to empathy) when

they heard the audios of individuals experiencing, than those that did not practice meditation.

Better memory

One of the reflections of the things has been connected to is boosting fast memory recall.

 Catherine Kerrl, a scientist at the Martinos Facility for Biomedical Imaging as well as the Osher Research Center, discovered that individuals who exercised conscious meditation could readjust the brain wave that screens out disturbances and also raise their performance faster that those that did not meditate.

 She stated that this capability to neglect distractions could discuss "their exceptional ability to swiftly remember and incorporate new realities.

" This seems to be extremely comparable to the power of being revealed to new scenarios that will also drastically improve our memory of points.

Much more noodle

Reflection has been connected to more substantial quantities of smarts in the hippocampus and frontal locations of the brain. I did not understand what this suggested initially; however, it ends up; it's pretty terrific.

 More gray matter can cause more positive emotions, longer-lasting emotional stability, and also heightened focus throughout everyday life.

Meditation has likewise been revealed to diminish age-related impacts on gray matter and also reduce the decrease of our cognitive performance.

Changes Frameworks in the Brain

Some research studies recommend exercising mindfulness reflection can change the structures of the brain.

A study published in the journal Psychiatry Research that was carried out by a team of scientists at Harvard College;
 made use of brain scans to determine that eight weeks of a mindfulness training program called Mindfulness-Based Anxiety Reduction (MBSR) increased the cortical thickness in the hippocampus, the part of the mind that manages discovering and memory as well as plays an important duty in emotion policy.

While scientists are still functioning to recognize the results of volume boosts or declines of the hippocampus, it is typically thought that boosts correlate to enhanced emotional law, while reductions are a risk factor for adverse feelings, like stress.

Furthermore, numerous mental wellness conditions, including significant depression and also trauma (PTSD), are associated with decreased volume and also density of the hippocampus.

The research study additionally located reductions in the quantity of the amygdala, the part of the brain involved with experiencing emotions like fear, stress, and anxiety, and anxiety.

What's even more, the observed brain changes matched the individuals' self-reporting of their degrees of stress and anxiety, indicating reflection not just altered frameworks in the mind, but exactly how those practicing it really felt.

A follow-up research study by the same scientists released in February 2014 in the journal Frontiers in Human Neuroscience additionally found that changes in the mind following reflection represented renovations in participants' regarded level of anxiety.

Stress Law

A small research study released in July 2016 in the journal Biological Psychiatry used brain scans to assess the effects of meditation on the brain and people's health.

For the research study, scientists hired 35 jobless grownups that were seeking employment and also were under a significant amount of stress.

The participants were taken into two teams for a three-day treatment: one that was educated an official program of mindfulness meditation and also one that was instructed a type of "phony" reflection program concentrating on distracting oneself from worries, such as with babble or jokes.

At the end of the intervention, participants undertook mind scans as well as located that those who had participated in the meditation training revealed extra meaningful tasks in the locations of the mind related to relaxing state.

At a follow up four months later, those that joined the meditation group also had reduced levels of a pen in their blood tied to harmful inflammation, a physical condition strictly about stress and anxiety.

Aids Improve Emphasis and Concentration

In today's busy world, with its numerous disturbances, everyone has difficulty maintaining emphasis once in a while. Possibly not remarkably, researchers say there's a factor to think that meditating can aid with that.

A research study published in March 2013 in the journal Psychological Science recommends that mindfulness meditation can decrease mind wandering as well as enhance cognitive performance.

The researchers located that a two-week mindfulness meditation program assisted individuals' emphasis as well as memory while finishing the GRE.

The training led to improved scores and also lowered the occurrence of sidetracked ideas.

Additional research, published in the Proceedings of the National Academy of Sciences, located comparable outcomes. Scientists compared the brains of experienced meditators to those of people new to the practice and paid precise focus to the default setting network (DMN), or the part of the brain that is active when the individual is not concentrated on the outdoors.

Basically, it's responsible for the wandering ideas that appear when you're sitting still or about to go to sleep.

The scientists discovered that in knowledgeable meditators, the DMN was fairly deactivated while the individuals were practicing various forms of reflection, which equates to fewer distracting thoughts than the beginner meditators.

Shield the Aging Mind

The preliminary research study likewise suggests that meditation may assist secure the mind against aging. A study released in the journal NeuroImage by a team from UCLA recommended that people that practice meditation has much less age-related degeneration in the brain's white matter.

Follow-Up research published in January 2015 in the journal Frontiers in Psychology discovered that meditation also shows up to assists the brain's smarts, the tissue that contains nerve cells, and is linked by the white matter.

For the study, the same scientists contrasted the brains of 50 people who had practiced meditation regularly over 20 years with the minds of those that did not.

People in both teams revealed a loss of grey brain issue as they aged, but for those that meditated, it decreased much less.

The researchers warned that the research could not draw a cause and effect partnership between meditation as well as protecting smarts in the brain.

Still, they say it is encouraging, as well as ask for even more study to additionally discover the practice's prospective safety benefits on the aging brain.

Easy methods to practice meditation

1. Discover a comfortably seated placement, preferably somewhere where you will not feel uneasy regarding anybody seeing you.

2. Soften your gaze or delicately shut your eyes.

3. Bring your focus to your breath, complying with each exhale, and breathe in for numerous full cycles.

4. Pay attention to the feeling of the breath, identifying a specific place in your body-- in your nostrils, at the rear of your ribs, under your sternum-- where the feeling feels pleasurable. Focus on that sensation as well as practice.

5. Carefully start to grin. Smile generally; however, without pressure. Do not develop tension in your face muscle mass. Smile as you would naturally, without even trying.

6. As thoughts arise, notice them, approve them, as well as let them go. Your brain might attempt to distract you by stating points like This is odd.
What am I doing? Or your mind might match your smile by offering a funny or satisfying idea, or it might oppose by stating something such as this is phony, I'm not satisfied. I'm upset about. Whatever your brain does, see it and then let it pass.

7. Preserve a steady, comfortable rhythm with your breath and keep a constant, gentle smile for the next couple of mins.

8. As you end this practice and also reenter your everyday routine, notification whether you grin faster or a lot more extensively. Notification whether you feel a little better, a little lighter, or even more certain

Brain Haze

What is brain haze?
Brain haze isn't a medical problem itself, however instead a sign of other medical conditions. It's a kind of cognitive disorder, including:
- memory problems
- absence of psychological clearness
- poor concentration
- lack of ability to concentrate
Some individuals likewise explain it as mental fatigue. Depending upon the intensity of mind fog, it can disrupt the job or school. Yet it doesn't need to be a permanent component in your life.

- Reasons.
- Medical diagnosis.
- Therapy.
- Expectation.

What are the sources of mind haze?
There are numerous descriptions of why mind haze takes place. When you identify the underlying cause, you can begin taking care of the issue. Right here are six possible reasons.
1. Stress
Persistent anxiety can increase high blood pressure, deteriorate the immune system, and activate clinical depression. It can likewise create psychological exhaustion.
When your mind is exhausted, it comes to be tougher to assume, factor, and also emphasis.
The impacts of stress on the body ".
2. Absence of rest
Poor sleep high quality can likewise disrupt just how well your brain functions. Go for 8 to 9 hrs of rest per evening. Sleeping too little can cause poor focus as well as gloomy ideas.
3. Reasons and danger elements for sleep problems
Hormonal modifications.

Hormone modifications can likewise activate brain haze. Stages of the hormones progesterone and estrogen grow during pregnancy. This change can impact memory and create short-term cognitive problems. Similarly, a decrease in estrogen degree throughout menopause can trigger lapse of memory, wrong concentration, and also gloomy thinking.

Discover the connection: Memory loss as well as menopause ".

4. Diet

Diet regimen can likewise play a role in mind haze. Vitamin B-12 supports a healthy and balanced mind feature, as well as a vitamin B-12 deficiency, which can bring about brain fog.

If you have food, allergic reactions, or sensitivities, brain haze might develop after consuming certain foods. Possible offenders consist of:

- MSG.

- aspartame.

- peanuts.

- dairy products.

Getting rid of trigger foods from your diet regimen may enhance symptoms.

5. Medications

If you see brain fog while taking the drug, talk with your physician. Mind fog might be a well-known side effect of the medication. Decreasing your dose or switching to another medicine may improve your symptoms.

Brain haze can also take place after cancer cell therapies. This is referred to as chemo brain.

6. Medical conditions

Clinical problems connected with inflammation, fatigue, or modifications in blood sugar levels can likewise trigger mental fatigue. For instance, mind haze is a symptom of fatigue syndrome, which involves persistent tiredness for longer than six or seven months.

Patients with fibromyalgia may suffer from the same haziness daily. Other problems that might trigger mind fog consist of:

- anemia.

- anxiety.

- diabetic issues.

- Sjogren disorder.

- migraines.
- Alzheimer's condition.
- hypothyroidism.
- autoimmune diseases such as lupus, arthritis, and numerous cases of sclerosis.
- dehydration.

How it's detected
See your doctor if you have a relentless lack of quality that intensifies or does not enhance. A single examination can't identify mind haze. Mind haze may signify an underlying concern, so your physician will certainly conduct a physical exam and also ask about your:
- psychological wellness.
- diet regimen.
- level of exercise.
- modern medicines or supplements.
You should allow your doctor to know about various other signs and symptoms you might have. As an example, someone with hypothyroidism may have brain haze together with loss of hair, dry skin, weight gain, or weak nails.
Blood work can assist your doctor in recognizing the source of mind fog. A blood examination can spot the following:
- irregular glucose levels.
- weak liver, kidney, and thyroid function.
- nutritional shortages.
- infections.
- inflammatory diseases.
Based on the results, your doctor will certainly determine whether to explore further.
 Other diagnostic tools may include imaging examinations to look inside the body, such as X-rays, MRI, or CT scans. The medical professional might likewise conduct allergic reaction screening or a sleep research to look for a rest condition.
Maintaining a food journal can aid you in figuring out if your diet regimen adds to brain haze.
Brain haze remedy.

Brain haze therapy depends upon what lead to it.

For example, if you're anemic, iron supplements may increase your production of red blood cells as well as minimize your mind haze.

If you're detected with an autoimmune condition, your medical professional might recommend a corticosteroid or various other medicine to lower swelling or reduce the immune system.

Sometimes, relieving brain haze is a matter of dealing with a dietary deficiency, switching over medicines, or enhancing the quality of your sleep.

Home remedies to boost mind haze include

- resting 8 to 9 hours per evening.
- managing tension by knowing your restrictions as well as preventing excessive alcohol and high levels of caffeine.
- exercising.
- enhancing your brainpower (shot volunteering or fixing brain puzzles).
- finding satisfying activities.
- raising your consumption of protein, fruits, vegetables, and also healthy and balanced fats.

The Relevance of Psychological Health And Fitness

- Mind-body connection.
- Advantages.
- Methods.
- Takeaway.

Keeping your mind in shape

Physical conditioning obtains lots of interest, as well as forever factor. A healthy and balanced body can prevent conditions such as illness and also diabetic issues and aid you preserve independence as you age. Mental health and fitness is just as essential as fitness, as well as should not be overlooked.

Consisting of psychological mastery exercises into your day-to-day regimen can assist you reap the benefits of a sharper mind and a healthier body for years ahead.

Psychological health and fitness indicate maintaining your brain as well as mental wellness in good shape. It does not show training for "mind Olympics" or acing an IQ test. It refers to a collection of exercises that assist you:

- reduce.
- unwind.
- improve a flagging memory.

Mind-body link

It's no surprise that the lot more you assist the body, the more you help your consciousness. The physical event increases the flow of oxygen to your account. It also increases the number of endorphins, the "feel-good" chemicals, in your brain.

Because of this, it's not unusual that individuals that are in excellent physical form also often tend to appreciate a higher degree of imagination.

Taking part in a strenuous physical exercise can assist you battle anxiety and get a much more positive outlook on life. It's also an excellent means to beat tension, which can harm you emotionally and literally.

Mental exercise is equally as useful. According to a study in the Procedures of the National Academy of Sciences, specific memory training workouts can raise "fluid intelligence," the ability to reason and address new troubles.

While exercise benefits the mind and also the body, so is meditation. Reflection, together with other approaches, is a different means to treat anxiety. Relaxing the mind permits you to problem solve in a much more relaxed ways.

Benefits of mental health and fitness

When you go to bed after a lengthy day, your body begins to loosen up. Yet the mind does not always comply with it.
Visualization can aid. You can often accomplish a feeling of serenity via images, the process of imagining a relaxing scene or place.
This method can decrease tension in both your body and also your consciousness by challenging neurons in the less-dominant area of your brain.
The less-dominant side of your brain is the location that manages sensations of a positive self-image and also a positive outlook.
When you think about something aside from your everyday concerns, you boost activity in the neural frameworks of that area of your mind.
Inevitably, visualization can improve your emotional wellness and tranquility you down mentally.

End up being emotionally fit
Keeping your mind mentally fit isn't as challenging as preparing for a marathon; however, it's a good analogy. You can add psychological exercises to the many tasks you already perform, such as:
- reading.
- fantasizing.
- searching for wit in life.
You may try the following methods to boost your mental health and fitness.
Quit multitasking
You might believe that multitasking enables you to obtain more points done at the same time, yet it creates even more problems than it resolves. Concentrating on one job at a time will boost your concentration as well as aid you in being more efficient.

Be positive with on your own
Favorable affirmation is one method of increased psychological proficiency.

Affirmation, or talking with on your own in a positive way, involves strengthening neural pathways to bring your self-esteem, well-being, and fulfillment to a higher level.

To start, make a listing of your top quality. Advise on your own that you don't have to be ideal. Establish objectives for what you wish to enhance and begin little to stay clear of ending up being overloaded.

Try something various

New experiences can additionally establish you on the course of psychological fitness. You can fit brand-new strategies right into your day-to-day life in a variety of means:

- Try brand-new foods.
- Attempt new ways to accomplish regular jobs.
- Travel to brand-new locations.
- Take a brand-new way to work or the food store.

According to the Alzheimer's Organization, a research study shows that maintaining your mind energetic increases its vitality. Doing brand-new things in new means shows up to retain brain cells as well as connections.

It may even produce new mind cells. Breaking out of your ordinary can help keep your brain stay healthy.

Play video games

Gamings that examine thinking and various other sections of your brain are fun methods to keep your mind sharp. Think about these video games:

- crossword challenges.
- parlor game.
- Sudoku.

Gamings are a fantastic means to build up your brain muscle. Also, busy action video games may improve your ability to learn new jobs, according to research in the journal Current Biology Trusted Resource. The research study located tentative evidence that video games may increase your focus period, response time, as well as task-switching ability.

 Along with computer games, try any kind of video game that uses making use of:.

- reasoning.
- thinking.

- trivia.
Find out more.
Reading is excellent for your brain. Also, as you're reading this sentence, your mind is processing each word, remembering the significance quickly.
Past the mechanics, reading assists, you picture the topic on the pages before you, as well as envision what voices sound like in the created dialogue. This can also be a fantastic leisure strategy.
Reading is a fantastic activity since it can stir the creative imagination and also ignite a lot of different parts of the brain. There are countless genres and even types of reviewing the material. It's unlikely that you'll lack fascinating things to check out.
Take the time
Psychological health and fitness don't need to take up a lot of your time. Investing a few mins on it can assist you really feel much better and also think even more clearly. Keep in mind that leisure and also visualization are equally as important in a mental workout as the much more energized tasks, such as memory exercises or game-playing. Try including 1 or 2 tasks each time to your mental activity, such as:
- relaxing.
- visualizing.
- verifying.
- memory workouts.
- game-playing.

The takeaway
Mental, physical fitness is essential to preserving your brain and also your body healthy, precisely as you age. There are lots of types of psychological mastery workouts, and also you do not require to head to the fitness center to do them.
They include energetic ones, such as discovering a brand-new tune or playing a video game, along with relaxed ones, such as relaxation and visualization workouts.
Schedule a mental health and fitness burglarize your schedule right alongside your workout routine. Your mind and your health and wellness deserve it.

11 Finest Foods to Boost Your Brain and Memory

Your brain is a big deal.

As the nerve center of your body, it supervises of maintaining your heart pounding and lungs breathing as well as enabling you to move, really feel as well as believe.

That's why it's an excellent idea to keep your mind in peak working problems.

The foods you eat contribute to maintaining your mind healthy and balanced and also can improve specific mental jobs, such as memory as well as concentration.

This post provides 11 foods that boost your mind.

1. Fatty Fish

When individuals talk about mind foods, oily fish is usually on top of the list.

This sort of fish includes salmon, trout, and also sardines, which are all abundant sources of omega-3 fats.

About 60% of your brain is made from fat, and also fifty percent of that fat is the omega-3 kind.

Your mind makes use of omega-3s to build brain and also afferent neurons, as well as these fats are essential for discovering as well as memory. Omega 3-s additionally have a couple of additional benefits for your mind.

For something, they may slow down age-related psychological decrease as well as aid ward off Alzheimer's illness. On the other side, not obtaining enough omega-3s is linked to finding out impairments, as well as anxiety.

In general, eating fish appears to have positive wellness benefits.

One research study found that individuals that ate baked or broiled fish had much more noodle in their minds. Gray matter contains a lot of the afferent neuron that controls decision making, memory as well as feeling.

On the whole, fatty fish is a superb choice for mental health.

Fatty fish is a precious resource of omega-3s, a significant foundation of the brain. Omega-3s contribute to developing memory and also improving mood, in addition to securing your mind versus the decrease.

2. Coffee

If coffee is the highlight of your early morning, you'll rejoice to hear that it benefits you.

Two main components in coffee-- high levels of caffeine and antioxidants-- assist your mind.

The high levels of caffeine in coffee have a variety of positive effects on the brain, consisting of:

- Increased awareness: High levels of caffeine keeps your mind alert by obstructing adenosine, a chemical carrier that makes you sleepy.

- Boosted state of mind: High levels of caffeine may additionally improve a few of your "feel-good" natural chemicals, such as serotonin.

- Sharp concentration: One research study discovered that when individuals consumed one large coffee in the early morning or smaller quantities throughout the day, they were more effective at jobs that required concentration.

Consuming alcohol coffee over the long term is also linked to a minimized risk of neurological conditions, such as Parkinson's as well as Alzheimer's.

This can a minimum of be partial as a result of coffee's high focus of antioxidants.

Coffee can assist boost alertness and also mood. It may also supply some security against Alzheimer's, thanks to its high levels of caffeine and also antioxidants.

3. Blueberries

Blueberries provide countless health and wellness advantages, including some that are specifically for your brain.

Blueberries and various other deeply colored berries provide anthocyanins, a group of plant compounds with anti-inflammatory as well as antioxidant impacts.

Anti-oxidants act versus both oxidative anxiety as well as inflammation, problems that may add to mind aging, and also neurodegenerative conditions.

A few of the antioxidants in blueberries have been located to collect in mind as well as help improve the interaction between brain cells.

Animal research studies have shown that blueberries aid boost memory and also may even postpone temporary memory loss. Attempt spraying them on your morning meal grain or including them to a smoothie.

Blueberries are packed with anti-oxidants that might postpone mind aging and also enhance memory.

4. Turmeric extract

Turmeric has created a great deal of buzz just recently.

This deep-yellow seasoning is a crucial component in curry powder as well as has a variety of advantages for the mind.

Curcumin, the active source in turmeric, has been shown to cross the blood-brain obstacle, indicating it can straight get in the mind and benefit the cells there.

It's a powerful antioxidant and also anti-inflammatory substance that has been linked to the adhering to brain advantages:

- Might benefit memory: Curcumin might help improve memory in people with Alzheimer's. It may also aid the removal of the amyloid plaques that are a trademark of this illness.

- Eases anxiety: It improves serotonin and dopamine, which both improve mood. One research study discovered curcumin boosted depression signs and symptoms just as high as an antidepressant over six weeks.

- Helps brand-new brain cells expand: Curcumin improves brain-derived neurotrophic aspect, a sort of development hormone that helps brain cells grow.

It might assist in delay age-related psychological decrease, yet more research study is required.

To profit from curcumin, try food preparation with curry powder, adding turmeric to potato recipes to transform them gold or making turmeric tea.

Turmeric and also its energetic substance curcumin have potent anti-inflammatory and antioxidant advantages, which help the mind. In research, it has minimized signs and symptoms of depression and Alzheimer's illness.

5. Broccoli

Broccoli is packed with active plant substances, including anti-oxidants.

It's also very high in vitamin K, delivering greater than 100% of the Recommended Daily Consumption (RDI) in a 1-cup (91-gram) offering.
This fat-soluble vitamin is crucial for developing sphingolipids, a type of fat that's densely packed into mind cells.
A few research studies in older adults have connected a higher vitamin K intake too much better memory. Past vitamin K, broccoli includes a variety of compounds that offer it anti-inflammatory and also antioxidant results, which might assist safeguard the brain against damage.
Broccoli contains several substances that have powerful anti-oxidant and also anti-inflammatory effects, including vitamin K.
6. Pumpkin Seeds
Pumpkin seeds have potent anti-oxidants that shield the body and mind from complimentary radical damage. They're additionally an excellent source of magnesium, iron, zinc as well as copper.
Each of these nutrients is important for mind wellness:
- Zinc: This element is critical for nerve signaling. Zinc deficiency has been connected to lots of neurological conditions, consisting of Alzheimer's illness, depression, and Parkinson's ailment. - Magnesium: Magnesium is crucial for learning and memory.
Low magnesium levels are linked to numerous neurological disease, consisting of migraine headaches, depression as well as epilepsy.
- Copper: Your mind makes use of copper to aid in regulating nerve signals. And also, when copper levels run out whack, there's a more significant threat of neurodegenerative problems, such as Alzheimer's.
- Iron: Iron shortage is frequently characterized by brain fog as well as damaged mind function.
The study focuses primarily on these micronutrients, instead of pumpkin seeds themselves. Nevertheless, considering that pumpkin seeds are high in these micronutrients, you can likely enjoy their benefits by adding pumpkin seeds to your diet plan.
Pumpkin seeds are abundant in lots of micronutrients that are very important for mind feature, including copper, iron, magnesium as well as zinc.

7. Dark Chocolate

Dark chocolate, as well as chocolate powder, are loaded with a few brain-boosting compounds, consisting of flavonoids, caffeine, and antioxidants.

Flavonoids are a set of antioxidant plant compounds.

The flavonoids in delicious chocolate collect in the areas of the brain that manage learning and also memory.

Researchers state these compounds might enhance memory and likewise assist decrease age-related psychological decrease. A number of researches back this up.

In one research,, including over 900 people, those who ate chocolate extra often carried out better in a collection of mental jobs, including some entailing memory, than those who seldom ate it.

Chocolate is also a legitimate mood booster, according to research.

One research study discovered that individuals who ate chocolate experienced increased favorable feelings compared to participants that ate biscuits.

Nonetheless, it's still unclear whether that's because of compounds in the delicious chocolate, or just because the scrumptious taste makes people satisfied.

The flavonoids in delicious chocolate may aid shield the mind. Research studies have recommended that consuming delicious chocolate can enhance both memory and mood.

8. Nuts

Research study has shown that consuming nuts can improve pens of heart wellness, as well as having a healthy and balanced heart is connected to having a healthy brain.

A 2014 evaluation revealed that nuts could improve cognition as well as also aid stop neurodegenerative illness. Likewise, one more big research discovered that females who consumed nuts regularly throughout numerous years had a sharper memory, contrasted to those who did not consume nuts.

Numerous nutrients in nuts, such as healthy fats, antioxidants, and also vitamin E, may clarify their brain-health benefits.

Vitamin E guards cell membrane layers against free radical damage, aiding slow psychological decline. While all nuts benefit your mind, walnuts may have an extra edge, since they likewise provide omega-3 fatty acids.

Nuts include a host of brain-boosting enriched, including vitamin E, healthy fats as well as plant substances.

9. Oranges

You can obtain all the vitamin C you need in a day by eating one tool orange.

Doing so is very important for brain wellness, considering that vitamin C is a crucial factor in protecting against mental decline. Consuming enough amounts of vitamin C-rich foods can secure against age-related psychological decrease and Alzheimer's disease, according to a 2014 review article.

Vitamin C is a powerful anti-oxidant that assists fight off the cost-free radicals that can damage mind cells. Plus, vitamin C supports brain health and wellness as you age.

You can likewise get superb amounts of vitamin C from bell peppers, guava, kiwi, tomatoes as well as strawberries.

Oranges, as well as various other foods that are high in vitamin C, can aid defend your brain against damages from complimentary radicals.

10. Eggs

Eggs are an excellent source of numerous nutrients linked to brain health, consisting of vitamins B6 and also B12, folate as well as choline (63).

Choline is a crucial trace element that your body uses to create acetyl-choline, a neurotransmitter that assists manage mood and memory.

Two research studies discovered that higher intakes of choline were linked to far better memory and mental function. Nonetheless, many people do not get enough choline in their diet regimen.

Consuming eggs is a straightforward way to obtain choline, considered that egg yolks are amongst the wealthiest resources of this nutrient. Appropriate intake of choline is 425 mg per day for most ladies as well as 550 mg daily for men, with merely a single egg yolk consisting of 112 mg.

Furthermore, the B vitamins have several functions in brain wellness. To begin, they might assist slow the progression of mental decrease in the senior.

Also, being deficient in two sorts of B vitamins-- folate and also B12-- has been connected to depression. Folate deficiency is common in elderly individuals with dementia, and also researches reveal that folic acid supplements can assist decrease age-related psychological decrease.

B12 is additionally involved in synthesizing brain chemicals and controlling sugar levels in the brain.

It's worth keeping in mind that there's a microscopic straight study on the web link between eating eggs and also brain health and wellness.

Nonetheless, there is research to sustain the brain-boosting advantages of the nutrients located in eggs.

Eggs are a rich source of different B vitamins and choline, which are very important for appropriate brain working and development, as well as managing state of mind.

11. Eco-friendly Tea

As holds with coffee, the caffeine in green tea boosts mind features.

It has been discovered to improve awareness, efficiency, memory as well as focus.

But green tea likewise has other parts that make it a brain-healthy beverage.

Among them is L-theanine, an amino acid that can go across the blood-brain obstacle and raise the task of the natural chemical GABA, which helps in reducing anxiousness as well as makes you feel more unwinded.

L-theanine likewise enhances the regularity of alpha waves in mind, which aids you to loosen up without making you feel worn out. One testimonial located that the L-theanine in environment-friendly tea can assist you to relax by combating the revitalizing impacts of high levels of caffeine.

It's likewise rich in polyphenols and also antioxidants that might shield the mind from mental decrease as well as lower the danger of Alzheimer's and Parkinson's.

Plus, environment-friendly tea has been found to improve memory.

Green tea is an outstanding drink to support your brain. Its high levels of caffeine web content improve alertness, while its anti-oxidants protect the brain, and L-theanine assists you unwind.

The 7 Worst Foods for Your Mind

Your brain is one of the most vital organs in your body.

It keeps your heart whipping, lungs breathing, and all the systems in your body working.

That's why it's crucial to maintain your brain operating in maximum condition with a healthy and balanced diet regimen.

Some foods have adverse results on the brain, affecting your memory and state of mind as well as raising your danger of dementia.

Quotes forecast that mental deterioration will positively impact more significant than 65 million people around the world by 2030.

Thankfully, you can help in reducing your danger of the illness by reducing specific foods out of your diet.

This post exposes the seven worst foods for your brain.

1. Sweet Drinks

Sugary beverages include beverages like soda, sports drinks, power drinks, and also fruit juice.

A high intake of sugary beverages not just increases your midsection as well as boosts your risk of kind two diabetes mellitus as well as a cardiovascular disease-- it additionally has an unfavorable result on your mind.

Too much intake of sugary drinks boosts the odds of establishing kind two diabetic issues, which has been revealed to increase the risk of Alzheimer's illness.

Additionally, higher sugar levels in the blood can raise the threat of mental deterioration, even in individuals without diabetes mellitus.

A key element of many sweet beverages is high-fructose corn syrup (HFCS), which consists of 55% fructose and 45% glucose.

High consumption of fructose can bring about obesity, high blood pressure, high blood fats, diabetic issues, and also arterial disorder. These aspects of metabolic syndrome may cause a boost in the long-lasting danger of developing dementia.

Animal researches have shown that high fructose intake can bring about insulin resistance in the brain, as well as a reduction in brain function, memory, discovering, and the development of mind nerve cells.

One research in rats located that a diet plan high in sugar increased brain swelling and impaired memory. Additionally, rats that took in a diet regimen consisting of 11% HFCS were worse than those whose diet plans contained 11% regular sugar.

One more study found that rats fed a high-fructose diet gained more weight, had even worse blood sugar level control, as well as a higher threat of metabolic problems as well as memory disabilities.

While refresher courses in human beings are required, the outcomes recommend that high consumption of fructose from sugary drinks might have additional unfavorable impacts on the brain, past the effects of sugar.

Some options to sugary drinks consist of water, bitter cold tea, veggie juice, as well as unsweetened dairy products.

High consumption of sweet drinks may raise the danger of dementia. High-fructose corn syrup (HFCS) may be specifically hazardous, creating brain inflammation and also impairing memory and knowing. Refresher courses in humans are needed.

2. Improved Carbs

Refined Carbohydrate consists of sugars and highly processed grains, such as white flour.

These kinds of carbs typically have a high glycemic index (GI). This indicates your body absorbs them rapidly, creating a spike in your blood glucose and insulin levels.

Additionally, when consumed in larger quantities, these foods often have a high glycemic ton (GL). The GL refers to just how much a food elevates your blood sugar levels, based upon the serving dimension. Foods that are high-GI, as well as high-GL, have been found to harm brain features.

A study has revealed that just a single meal with high glycemic lots can harm memory in both children as well as an adult.

Another research in healthy and balanced university students discovered that those that had a higher intake of fat and polished sugar additionally had imperfect memory.

This effect on memory might be due to swelling of the hippocampus, a part of the mind that affects some elements of consciousness, as well as responsiveness to hunger and fullness cues.

Inflammation is acknowledged as a risk aspect for degenerative diseases of the brain, including Alzheimer's disease and dementia.

For example, one research study took a look at senior people that took in more than 58% of their daily calories in the form of carbs. The research discovered they had nearly dual the danger of moderate psychological problems and also mental deterioration.

Carbs might have many other results on the brain too. As an example, one study discovered that kids aged 6 to 7 who consumed diet regimens high in polished carbohydrates likewise racked up reduced on nonverbal intelligence.

Nevertheless, this research could not determine whether eating polished carbohydrates created these lower scores, or merely whether the two variables were related.

Healthy and balanced, lower-GI carbohydrates include foods such as veggies, fruits, beans as well as entire grains. You can utilize this data source to discover the GI as well as GL of common foods.

A high intake of polished carbohydrates with a high glycemic index (GI) and glycemic tons (GL) may harm memory and also intelligence, along with increase the danger of mental deterioration. These consist of sugars and very processed grains like white flour.

3. Foods High in Trans Fats

Trans fats are a sort of unsaturated fat that can have a detrimental effect on brain health and wellness.

While trans fats take place naturally in animal products like meat as well as dairy, these are not a significant problem. It's industrially produced trans fats, also called hydrogenated vegetable oils, that are an issue.

These artificial trans fats can be found in reducing margarine, icing, junk food, ready-made cakes, and also packaged cookies.

Research studies have discovered that when people take in higher quantities of trans fats, they often tend to have an increased threat of Alzheimer's condition, more imperfect memory, lower mind volume, and also cognitive decrease.

4However, some research studies have not found an association between trans-fat consumption and even brain health and wellness. However, trans fats must be prevented.

They hurt numerous various other elements of health and wellness, consisting of heart health and wellness and also swelling.

The evidence on saturated fat is blended. Three observational research studies have discovered a favorable association between saturated fat intake and also the threat of Alzheimer's condition, whereas a fourth study revealed the contrary effect.

One reason for this may be that a part of the test populations had a genetic vulnerability to the condition, which is triggered by a gene referred to as ApoE4. However, more research study is required on this subject.

One research of 38 ladies found that those that ate more hydrogenated fat relative to unsaturated fat executed even worse on memory and also acknowledgment procedures.

Thus, it might be that the loved one ratios of fat in the diet regimen are a vital aspect, not just the type of fat itself.

For instance, diets high in omega-3 fats have been discovered to aid shield against the cognitive decrease. Omega-3s boost the secretion of anti-inflammatory compounds in the brain as well as can have a safety impact, particularly in older grownups.

You can raise the quantity of omega-3 fats in your diet plan by eating foods like fish, chia seeds, flax seeds, and walnuts.

Trans fats might be associated with damaged memory and the risk of Alzheimer's, but the proof is mixed. Removing trans fats entirely and also boosting the unsaturated fats in your diet regimen might be a great technique.

4. Very Processed Foods

Very refined foods often tend to be high in sugar, included fats and also salt.

They include foods such as chips, desserts, instant noodles, microwave popcorn, store-bought sauces, as well as ready-made dishes.

These foods are generally high in calories and reduced in various other nutrients. They're precisely the type of foods that trigger weight gain, which can hurt your brain health and wellness.

Research in 243 individuals discovered enhanced fat around the organs, or natural fat, is associated with brain cells damages. An additional research study in 130 people found there's a measurable decline in brain cells also at the beginning of metabolic syndrome.

The nutrient composition of processed foods in the Western diet regimen can likewise adversely influence the mind and add to the advancement of degenerative illness.

A study consisting of 52 individuals located that a diet regimen high in harmful ingredients caused lower degrees of sugar metabolism in the brain and a decrease in mind tissue. These aspects are thought to be markers for Alzheimer's condition.

An additional study, including 18,080 individuals, discovered that a diet regimen high in deep-fried foods, as well as processed meats, is related to reduced scores in identifying as well as memory.

Comparable outcomes were discovered in one more large-scale research in 5,038 individuals. A diet high in red meat, processed meat, baked beans as well as fried food was related to inflammation as well as a faster decline in reasoning over one decade.

In animal researches, rats fed a high-fat, high-sugar diet for eight months revealed impaired learning ability and negative adjustments to mind plasticity.

One more study discovered that rats fed a high-calorie diet experienced disruptions to the blood-brain obstacle.

The blood-brain barrier is a membrane layer between the brain and blood supply for the remainder of the body. It protects the brain by stopping some compounds from entering.

One of the ways refined foods may adversely influence the brain is by reducing the production of a molecule called brain-derived neurotrophic factor (BDNF).

This molecule is located in various parts of the mind, including the hippocampus, as well as it is crucial for a lasting memory, finding out and the growth of new nerve cells.

Consequently, any reduction can have a negative influence on these functions.

You can stay clear of refined foods by consuming primarily fresh, whole grains such as fruits, veggies, nuts, seeds, vegetables, meat, and also fish. Besides, a Mediterranean-style diet regimen has been revealed to secure against the cognitive decrease.

Refined foods add to excess fat around the body organs, which is connected with a decline in mind tissue. Besides, Western-style diet plans may increase brain swelling as well as impair memory, finding out, mind plasticity and the blood-brain barrier.S

5. Aspartame

Aspartame is a sweetening agent made use of in several sugar-free products.

People frequently pick to use it when trying to slim down or stay clear of sugar when they have diabetes mellitus. It is also located in numerous industrial items not explicitly targeted at individuals with diabetes mellitus.

Nonetheless, this commonly made use of sugar has also been connected to behavioral and cognitive problems, though the research study has been controversial.

Aspartame is made of phenylalanine, methanol, and also aspartic acid. Phenylalanine can go across the blood-brain barrier and also could interfere with the production of natural chemicals. Furthermore, aspartame is a chemical stress factor as well as might raise the mind's susceptibility to oxidative tension.

Some researchers have suggested these aspects may trigger adverse results on learning and feelings, which have been observed when aspartame is consumed in excess.

One research took a look at the results of a high-aspartame diet plan. Participants consumed regarding 11 mg of aspartame for every single extra pound of their body weight (25 mg per kg) for eight days.

By the end of the study, they were much more cranky, had a higher rate of anxiety, and carried out worse on psychological examinations.

One more research study found individuals who consumed synthetically sweetened sodas had an increased danger of stroke and dementia actually, though the specific type of sugar was not specified.

Some speculative research studies in mice and also rats have likewise supported these searchings.

Research of repeated aspartame intake in mice found that it hindered memory and also raised oxidative anxiety in the brain. One more found that long-term consumption caused inequality in antioxidant conditions in mind.

Various other pet experiments have not found any unfavorable impacts, though these were commonly large, single-dose experiments instead of long-term ones. Furthermore, mice and rats are supposedly 60 times much less conscious phenylalanine than humans.

Despite these searchings for, aspartame is still taken into consideration to be a safe sugar total if people eat it at regarding 18-- 23 mg per pound (40-- 50 mg per kg) of body weight per day or much less. According to these standards, a 150-pound (68-kg) individual ought to keep their aspartame intake under concerning 3,400 mg each day, at the maximum.

For referral, a package of sweetener consists of about 35 mg of aspartame, and a regular 12-ounce (340-ml) can of diet soda has concerning 180 mg. Quantities may differ depending on the brand.

Furthermore, several documents have reported that aspartame has no adverse effects.

Nonetheless, if you 'd like to avoid it, you might simply cut artificial sweeteners and excess sugar from your diet plan altogether.

Aspartame is a sweetening agent discovered in numerous soft drinks and sugar-free products. It has been connected to behavioral and also cognitive troubles, though generally it is thought about a risk-free product.

6. Alcohol

When consumed in small amounts, alcohol can be a pleasurable addition to a great meal. Nevertheless, excessive consumption can have severe effects on the brain.

Chronic alcohol usage results in a reduction in brain volume, metabolic modifications as well as disruption of natural chemicals, which are chemicals the mind utilizes to interact.

Individuals with alcoholism commonly have a deficiency in vitamin B1; this can result in a brain condition called Wernicke's encephalopathy, which consequently can turn into Korsakoff's disorder.

This disorder is identified by severe damage to the mind, consisting of memory loss, disruptions in vision, complication, and also unsteadiness.

Excessive usage of alcohol can additionally have unfavorable effects in non-alcoholics.

Hefty one-off alcohol consumption episodes are called "binge drinking." These severe episodes can cause the brain to interpret psychological hints in a different way than regular. For example, individuals have a decreased sensitivity to long faces and also an enhanced level of sensitivity to upset faces.

It's thought that these modifications to emotion acknowledgment might be a reason for alcohol-related aggressiveness.

Additionally, alcohol consumption during pregnancy can have destructive impacts on the fetus. Considered that its mind is still developing, the toxic results of alcohol can lead to developmental problems like fetal alcohol disorder.

The impact of alcoholic abuse in teenagers can additionally be particularly destructive, as the brain is still creating. Teens who drink alcohol have irregularities in brain structure, feature, and also behavior, compared to those that do not.

Notably, alcohol blended with energy beverages is worrying. They cause enhanced prices of binge alcohol consumption, damaged driving, dangerous habits as well as a raised danger of alcohol dependence.

An added result of alcohol is the disturbance of sleep patterns. Consuming a massive quantity of alcohol before bed is related to inadequate sleep top quality, which can lead to chronic sleep deprivation.

However, modest alcohol consumption may have beneficial results, including improved heart health as well as a minimized danger of diabetes. These practical effects have been mainly kept in mind in moderate wine consumption of one glass per.

Generally, you need to prevent extreme alcohol usage, particularly if you're a young adult or young person, as well as prevent binge drinking completely.

If you are pregnant, it is best to prevent alcohol consumption from alcohol altogether.

While modest alcohol consumption can have some favorable health impacts, excessive usage can bring about memory loss, behavior adjustments, and also sleep disruption. Particularly risky teams include young adults, young adults as well as expectant women.

7. Fish High in Mercury

Mercury is a heavy metal impurity and also the neurological poison that can be kept for a long time in animal cells.

Long-lived, the predatory fish, are especially vulnerable to building up mercury and can carry quantities over 1 million times the concentration of their surrounding water.

Therefore, the central food resource of mercury in human beings is seafood, especially wide ranges.

After a person consumes mercury, it spreads throughout their body, focusing in the brain, liver as well as kidneys. In expectant females, it additionally concentrates in the placenta and also the unborn child.

The effects of mercury toxicity consist of interruption of the central nervous system and neurotransmitters and stimulation of neurotoxins, resulting in damage to the mind.

For developing fetuses as well as kids, mercury can interfere with brain development and trigger the damage of cell elements. This can lead to spastic paralysis, as well as various other developmental delays as well as deficits.

Nonetheless, the majority of fish are not a substantial resource of mercury. Fish is a high-quality protein as well as has several vital nutrients, such as omega-3s, vitamin B12, zinc, iron, and magnesium. For that reason, it is essential to consist of fish as part of a healthy and balanced diet plan.

Commonly, it is suggested that grownups eat two to three servings of fish weekly. Nonetheless, if you're consuming shark or swordfish, only eat one offering, and after that, nothing else fish that week.

Expectant females and youngsters ought to prevent or restrict high-mercury fish, consisting of shark, swordfish, tuna, orange approximately, king mackerel, and tilefish. Nonetheless, it's still secure to have two to three servings of other low-mercury fish per week.

Recommendations may differ from nation to country, depending on the kinds of fish in your area, so it's always best to talk to your local food security agency for the recommendations that are right for you. Likewise, if you are capturing your fish, it is a great suggestion to contact neighborhood authorities regarding the levels of mercury in the water you are fishing from.

Mercury is a neurotoxic aspect that can be specifically harmful to developing fetuses and also children. The principal source in the diet regimen is big predatory fish such as shark and swordfish. It is best to limit your consumption of fish that are high in mercury.

The Bottom Line

Your diet plan most definitely has a substantial effect on your brain health.

Inflammatory diet regimen patterns that are high in sugar, improved carbs, undesirable fats as well as refined foods can contribute to impaired memory and also learning, as well as raise your danger of conditions such as Alzheimer's and mental deterioration.

Several other materials in food are dangerous for your mind as well. Alcohol can cause substantial damages to the mind when consumed in significant amounts, while mercury discovered in fish and shellfish can be neurotoxic as well as permanently damage, creating thoughts. Nevertheless, this doesn't mean you must prevent all these foods entirely. Some foods like alcohol and also fish also have health advantages.

Brain Vitamins: Can Vitamins Boost Memory?

- Vitamin B-12
- Vitamin E.
- Other prospective remedies.
- Best methods.
- Way of life choices that damage memory.

Whether you struggle with Alzheimer's disease or you have memory troubles, particular vitamins and also fatty acids have been stated to slow down or stop memory loss. The lengthy list of prospective solutions includes vitamins like vitamin B-12, natural supplements such as ginkgo Biloba, and omega-3 fats. But can a tablet increase your memory?

Much of the evidence for the preferred "remedies" aren't solid. Here, we discuss what recent professional researches need to claim about vitamins as well as amnesia.

Vitamin B-12

Scientists have long been looking into the partnership in between reduced degrees of B-12 (cobalamin) and memory loss. According to a Mayo Center specialist, having sufficient B-12 in your diet regimen can enhance memory. Nonetheless, if you get an adequate amount of B-12, there is no evidence that higher intake has positive effects. The promising study does show that B-12 can slow down cognitive decline in people with early Alzheimer's when taken together with omega-3 fatty acids.

B-12 shortage is most common in individuals with digestive tract or belly concerns, or stringent vegetarians. The diabetic issues drug metformin has likewise been revealed to lower B-12 degrees.

You must have the ability to obtain sufficient B-12 usually, as it's found in foods such as fish and fowl. Fortified morning meal cereal is an excellent choice for vegetarians.

Vitamin E

There is some proof to recommend that vitamin E can benefit the mind and also memory in older individuals. A 2014 Trusted Resource in

JAMA: The Journal of the American Medical Association discovered that high amounts of vitamin E could assist people with moderate to moderate Alzheimer's illness.

Individuals took doses of 2,000 worldwide systems (IU) a day. However, this quantity is not safe, according to Dr. Gad Marshall of Harvard Medical School.

Taking more than 1,000 IU a day is specifically dangerous for people with heart disease, particula

rly for those on blood thinners. It additionally increases the danger of prostate cancer.

Despite your age or condition, you need to be able to obtain sufficient vitamin E from your food. Ask your physician if you have an interest in added amounts.

Vitamin E shortage is uncommon, although it might take place in people on low-fat diet plans.

The vitamin is found in:

- nuts.

- seeds.

- dark-colored fruits, such as blueberries, avocados, and blackberries.

- vegetables, such as spinach as well as bell peppers.

Other possible treatments

When talking of ginkgo Biloba, both older and also further recent research Relied on Resource concur: The supplement does not seem to slow down memory loss or prevent the risk of Alzheimer's illness.

There isn't much evidence to suggest a connection between omega-3 and memory, either. Nonetheless, the study is presently in progress.

One recent research study published in the journal Alzheimer's & Dementia showed that fish oil could enhance non-Alzheimer's- associated brain handling.

Study results revealed that people who took fish oil supplements had much less mind atrophy than those that really did not.

Another research Relied on Source entailing healthy adults between the ages of 18 and 45 years revealed that taking 1.16 grams a day of docosahexaenoic acid (DHA) assisted in speeding up response time in short-term memory. Nevertheless, while reaction time boosted, consciousness itself didn't.

DHA is one main sort of omega-3 fatty acid, and also EPA (eicosapen-taenoic acid) is another. You can find them usually in body organ meats and even fish such as salmon.

Most excellent means to help your memory

For young and older people alike, it's valuable to get your dietary vitamins from the food you consume. Supplements can fill out the gaps but talk to your medical professional before you look at the recommended day-to-day consumption.

No matter your age, the most effective means to combat memory decline is to eat well and also exercise your body in addition to your mind, recommends Marshall. He very suggests the Mediterranean diet regimen as an excellent source of all the vitamins your body demands.

The Mediterranean diet regimen has been citeTrusted Source as a method to improve memory. The trademarks of the diet include:

- mostly plant-based foods.

- restricting (or eliminating) red meat.

- consuming fish.

- utilizing liberal quantities of olive oil to prepare dishes.

Find out more: The Mediterranean diet plan: 21 dishes ".

Diet plans that are similar to the Mediterranean diet consist of the MIND diet plan along with the DASHBOARD (dietary techniques to stop hypertension) diet plan. Both diets Trusted Resource had been located to lower the incidence of Alzheimer's disease.

The MIND diet, in particular, emphasizes the intake of green, leafed vegetables and plant-based food along with the high healthy protein as well as olive oil recommendations of the Mediterranean diet plan.

Having a strong support network and also being participated in your local neighborhood have been suggested as a means to postpone or protect against mental deterioration. Developing healthy and balanced rest behaviors can additionally protect your mind

. Research studies Trusted Source continues to confirm that routine exercise triggers the brain in manner ins which various other leisure activities do not. This can cause enhanced memory and cognitive feature over the long term.

Lifestyle selections that hurt memory

You can start to take care of your brain by merely being even more mindful of foods and routines that have been revealed to damage the brain. Fried food has been connected to the cardiovascular system damage Trusted Source, which affects the performance of the mind. Fried food likewise results in high cholesterol degrees, and also research study has attached mental deterioration to high cholesterol. Many Alzheimer's threat aspects, such as obesity as well as a sedentary way of living, are in your control. Also, altering one of these risk elements has been shown to Trusted Resource hold-up the onset of mental deterioration.

Why Our Minds Feel SO Taxed

When our mind is misused, the resultant result is that we would certainly begin to feel worn down in addition to losing focus.

Have you ever before asked yourself why you are not able to get most of your jobs finished? It could be that you are utilizing your brain the wrong way!

I lately started the study of just how my mind resolves the eyes of David Rock, the author of the book "Your Mind at the workplace," and I am learning a lot.

Today, I would be sharing some of the surprises I found out about my brain and things I can do to improve.

Shocks
1. Mindful thinking entails deeply intricate biological interactions in mind among billions of nerve cells.

2. Every time the mind works with a suggestion knowingly, it uses up a measurable and also minimal source.

3. Some psychological processes occupy a great deal much more energy than others, which is why one feels exhausted and tired after a particular mental exercise.

4. The most crucial mental processes, such as focusing on, usually take one of the most efforts. I can see why preparation takes up so much time in enhancement to depleting one's mind power.

The complying with points can help in getting rid of these difficulties:
1. Consider conscious thinking as a valuable source to preserve.
2. Focus on focusing on, as

it's an energy-intensive activity.
3. Save psychological power for focusing on by staying clear of other high-energy-consuming conscious tasks such as dealing with e-mails.
4. Set up one of the most attention-rich tasks when you have a fresh and also sharp mind.
5. Use the brain to communicate with information as opposed to attempting to store details, by producing visuals for complicated concepts and also by noting tasks.
6. Schedule blocks of time for various modes of thinking.
Put these lessons in practice throughout today and also share your responses in the comments section. I would enjoy reading exactly how you really felt applying them.

10 Smart Tips to Prevent Interruptions and Own Your Emphasis

Whatever sort of work you're doing, you're possibly dealing with some distraction-- whether it's digital, personally, or inner.

Your capacity to remain concentrated is higher than merely a beneficial thing to cultivate-- it's a critical consideration of your success or failure. Obtaining points done is necessary, and the emphasis is the key to getting points are done.

Right here are ten pointers to aid you to remain concentrated at the office by handling distraction, drawing healthy and balanced limits, and also eliminating chances for laziness:

1. Look into yourself

Interruptions can be internal along with external, so begin by looking within. If you're all over the place, ask yourself what's taking place. What's the source of your flightiness or stress and anxiety? What do you need to be working within your life?

2. Pinpoint the cause

As soon as you have your internal priorities ironed out, take a look at more external reasons. Is it your office setup? An intrusive colleague? An absence of ability, ideas, or time for something you require to be doing? Fatigue? When you can identify the reason, you can fix the result.

3. Be prepared

All successful leaders are terrific organizers; they make listings for every single significant and minor objective. When a job comes to your method, invest a long time thinking about just how you will accomplish it.

 Jot down every step needed throughout, with a timeline (even if it's a harsh one). There is a saying that every 10 mins you invest in planning conserve an hour in execution.

4. Go offline

Several of the most extensive resources of distraction originated from email, social media sites, as well as mobile phones. If you desire real emphasis, take yourself offline till you've completed what you need to do.

5. Offer yourself a break

One of the secrets to doing great work is to know when to relax. When you begin to feel distracted, take a break, and afterward reassess as well as redouble on your own. It does not merely act as an incentive-- a short break can aid your mind come to be more precise.

6. Tune it out

One of the very best means to tune everything out is to tune in to music. When everything around you is sidetracking, put on your headphones-- find something that can work as background music as opposed to music that holds your full focus. Songs can help you focus, and also the headphones signal others that you're not readily available to the conversation.

7. Break it down

Specifically, when interruptions are high, make jobs smaller sized and break down your big tasks right into smaller tasks to assist you to concentrate and offer you a feeling of achievement and also development.

8. Clean it up

What's the state of your office or workspace? If it's filthy, messy, or messy, spend a long time in removing it out so you can concentrate.

9. Set a deadline

If you're dealing with a complicated job, it takes approximately 90 mins to achieve anything rewarding-- and regarding 30 minutes to obtain your mind on the job.

As soon as you are in the flow, established a focused period -- as well as when the moment goes out, stop. It's less complicated to remain focused when you have an end visible.

10. End up being an early bird

This is a simple thing, but the benefits are terrific if you can pull it off: Start your day an hour before everybody else. Use that hr to organize your day and also to get going before there are any disturbances. Similarly, avoid the lengthy workplace lunches most days and also instead provide yourself a time-out to take a walk or clear your head, with something light and too nutritious to keep your blood glucose consistent. You'reoffering yourself time and energy.

The diversions that surround us aren't going anywhere, so learning to conquer them is just one of the best things you can do on your own. Offer some of these suggestions a shot, and let me recognize if you're feeling much more reliable and also less distracted.

An Easy Guide to Vacant Your Mind

" Empty your mind, be formless, unformed - like water. Now you place water into a cup, it comes to be the cup, you placed water right into a bottle, it ends up being the bottle, you put it in a teapot, it becomes the teapot.
 Now water can stream, or it can crash. Be water, my friend." ~ Bruce Lee

A lot of us think that our mind is designed to host a consistent stream of ideas, and there is nothing we can do concerning it. The mind supervises as well as we comply with. The humming can not stop, and also we can not make it quit.

Your mind is a device that you can manage-- if you select to. It can be an asset that allows you to experience beautiful things. It can likewise be a source of pain and misery if you let it obsess on adverse thoughts such as fear and all its symptoms.

The cycle
An untamed mind lives on feeding the same ideas and also generating the very same experiences. A typical period is something like this.
You might ask, what's wrong with this cycle. There is absolutely nothing incorrect with it if you're feeling excellent and also experiencing what brings you joy.
Nonetheless, if you're responding based on unfavorable thoughts and also limiting beliefs, you won't have control as well as you will adversely react to the majority of the moment.
The mind tends to stay much more on the unfavorable than favorable.

Break the cycle
To clear your mind is to release what's taking precious area in your mind and heart that's not offering you.
As soon as you refine what's on your mind, you gain viewpoint. You act, when required, from quality as well as truth. You no longer feed the loop.
An empty mind is:
- Conscious-- embracing the here and now minute and also experience

- Serene-- it doesn't harp on the same thoughts
- Intuitive-- it's responsive of input from more considerable resources
- Free-- from judgment and also fear
- Imaginative-- permitting inspiration as well as new ideas ahead in
- Loosened up-- it releases stress and also cultivates wellness
- Invigorated-- no effort is lost on undesirable thoughts

How To Make The Mind Unlimited

The ordinary human mind, while it functions all the time, works at a superficial level, unless boosted and trained. Educating your brain to operate at peak effectiveness raises your efficiency, help your capability to find out new info, and also stirs the imaginative juices.

While it is a misconception that people utilize just ten percent of their mental ability, indeed, lots of people's minds are not functioning at peak effectiveness.

Nevertheless, you can change that and also educate your mind to be extra absorbent, more imaginative, and more productive.

Frequently, individuals, when confronted with trouble, get on confusion as well as irritation. Once they learn exactly how to train their brains, the ability to change to logic and also quality becomes a force of habit.

Your mind can help extreme focus; you require to develop the capability to concentrate on an issue.

The excellent thinkers of our culture have discovered this trick. As soon as learned, you will certainly not fall into the emotional catch of confusion and aggravation anymore, and also you'll recognize just how to focus quickly on the trouble and the service you need.

Thanks to the research study, scientists have discovered that it is feasible for you to find out to re-shape your brain, only by changing your thoughts and emotions. They located that certain sorts of meditation made it possible to enhance the activity of the prefrontal cortex.

They discovered a means to raise mental activity without necessarily enhancing adrenaline and also stress. Their research found that concentrating on positive thoughts and feelings gave an enormous increase in brain tasks.

This does not indicate you require to chant a rule or go to your pleased location while practicing meditation.

The scientists found that merely believing satisfied; loving thoughts make your brain go into overtime, making psychological connections and also being active as well as innovative.

Whether you've been learned reflection methods or not, you can learn to boost your mind's activity, without stress and anxiety.

For starters, offer on your own only ten minutes in the early morning and also ten mins at night to focus on satisfied, caring ideas. Transforming the means you believe and depends on you.

Henry Ford stated, "If you assume you can do a thing or think you can't do something, you're right.

" Discover a comfy place to rest, kick back and also take a deep breath with your nose. Close your eyes and concentrate initially on your breathing. After that, focus on thinking of being joyous.

Brush aside the concerns and also focus on nothing by pleasure, happiness, and love.

You can transform the means your mind functions, but it takes discipline, resolution as well as method. If you wish to be smarter, you have to pick to do so, by managing your ideas as well as feelings - by choosing to be pleased, grateful, as well as satisfied.

By selecting to be mentally happy, you are altering the method your brain functions, making brand-new connections, actually rewiring your brain to be much more productive, much more imaginative, and also smarter.

I know you're asking, why just making yourself feel happy can perhaps have anything to do with obtaining smarter. It's basic. When your body feels good, blood flows through the brain smoothly.

This assists you to focus as well as lets your mind be as creative as it requires to be for the job available.

Happiness releases hormonal agents and body chemicals that will undoubtedly create the most magnificent mental task. Clinical depression and worry congest the works, making your psychological responsibility slow to a crawl and developing a slowness in the blood circulation as well as assumed processes.

There suffices mental confusion being thrown at you from all instructions, the last point you require is to be pounded by contradictory ideas and emotions.

All the fears as well as upsets, frustrations as well as anxiousness simply wipes out the discovering process.

When you're distressed as well as confused, it's hard to bear in mind points, or perhaps believe directly. Also, your observational skills are hindered by negativity as well as psychological upheaval. You can not enhance your brain while under the attack of fears and anxiousness. That's why the ten-minute two times a day are so crucial to your brain. Throughout those times, you should not allow any negativeness into your consciousness.

Permit your mind to loosen up with positive, kind, loving, pleased ideas. Think of all that you're grateful for in your life, every little thing that makes you satisfied.

Push aside any fears and also upsets, at least for that twenty mins a day. It's particularly important to begin your day feeling pleased and unwinded to survive your workday, and also, it's similarly essential to finish the day with those satisfying feelings to assist you to sleep comfortably, undisturbed every day's events, whether good or bad.

Rejoicing minimizes the complication in your mind, unwinding your brain as well as your body and enabling creativity and also psychological quality to keep you on the path. This assists the psychological links in your mind to remain transparent as well as sensible.

Due to the battle or trip hormonal agents swamping our system, we tend to make choices based on concern. Instead of dealing with the fears and also working through them, we make choices to assist us in staying clear of discomfort and even confusion

. However, that works against us rather than for us. Our brains inform us to prevent anything that can harm us. That includes not just physical damage, yet humiliation, shame, loss of respect and also credibility by peers, even loss of love. As a result, in anxiety, we make wrong selections, delay modifications that would assist us, and also attempt to stay clear of any risk in any way.

Basing agreement on fear never works in your support. It merely keeps you from completely living life, and as a matter of fact, can suppress the understanding and also growing process that maintains us alive and also keeps our brains healthy.

After you grasp the ability to educate your mind to work for you, as opposed to against you, it's time to begin obtaining that brain in shape. You exercise your body, why not your mind also? You understand that using your body makes you feel great and also improves your life as well as enhances longevity. Consequently, it's time to give your mind a good workout.

Believe it or not, among the methods you can extend your brain's muscle mass is by playing video games. That's right; I said computer game. Playing the games does provide your mind with moderate exercise.

It allows you to create your peripheral vision, something exceptionally useful in the real-life too. It likewise educates you to acknowledge duplicating patterns and also to keep in mind details, also beneficial in the real life. You're also finding out with each video game you understand. For those that belief playing a computer game is just for nerds and nerds, there is, in fact, a large neighborhood of people who delight in the obstacle of these games and also are bent on understanding the abilities.

Several are video games of approach, as well as beneficial for teaching your brain. In most of the games, working your way via the numerous degrees is much like functioning your means with the degrees of real life, discovering as you go.

Those who oppose the concept of computer game being instructional say that the games are violent, that they are addictive and time-consuming, and that young people especially are wasting their time.

Just like anything in life, possibly small amounts requires to be applied. On the bonus side, playing the games enables us to learn and get rid of challenges, which is an advantage.

Never quit discovering, growing, and also being innovative. It benefits your brain.

An additional method to stretch your mind is to reveal it to new ideas. Discover new locations of understanding. Even if you've never agreed with a suggestion, it does not imply you can not provide it some insight.

Stretch it a little to consist of some new truths. Avoid entering a rut and also coming to be set in your methods.

Have a specific interest in your life, something that gives you incredible pleasure. Locate a team of like-minded people, a club, if you will. It can be in your regional area or online. The point is to have some fascinating conversations, some exchange, trading info, and also concepts.

That will undoubtedly stretch your mind and make you feel good as well as your account boosted. Try signing up with a book club to review some great fiction. An excellent story will catch your passion, pull you in and allow you learn more about the personalities. Can not locate a book club? Begin one!

An additional method to relax as well as permit your mind to stretch is by paying attention to songs. Researchers claim that music can help you think better as well as enhance your mental capacity.

 At UC Irvine's Facility for Neurobiology of Knowing as well as Memory, a study was done on songs and also precisely how it affects the brain. Thirty-six pupils were given the standard spatial examinations located in I.Q. tests. Before the test, they were listened to Mozart's sonata for 2 Pianos in D Major for 10 minutes.

 They paid attention to leisure tapes before the 2nd examination and merely sat in silence before the third examination.

 All the pupils did incredibly better after listening to Mozart. They averaged 9 I.Q. points greater after listening to the songs.

The music put the students into a receptive state of mind for the tests, so they carried out, in reality, to have much better access to the sources in their minds.

Those entailed with songs regularly are better at fixing issues and also when checked, scored eighty percent more than those not in a music program.

 If trouble resolving becomes part of your daily life, and that holds for everyone, then let the music play.

Your Conscious & Your Subconscious

When it comes to mental capacity, your mindful mind is just one-sixth of your brain's reasoning ability. Nonetheless, your subconscious represents five-sixths of that ability.

That indicates that assembled, and your entire account has sufficient power to resolve any problem that comes your way.

Your mindful mind can hold seven items of details in the temporary memory; however, your subconscious mind shops every bit of understanding you have ever learned.

It consists of whatever you have actually ever listened to, believed, read, or even pictured.

Actually, you are much smarter than you think you are, thanks to the amazing memory of your subconscious mind. It's from the subconscious mind that authors and musicians obtain their ideas.

"The intelligence has little to do when traveling to exploration. There comes a leap in the mind, call it instinct or what you will, and the service concerns you, and also you don't know just how or why," said Albert Einstein. This is the work of your subconscious.

The most effective part regarding your subconscious is that you can set it to work on whatever trouble you're dealing with and also it will certainly function continuously, night and day, even while you're sleeping. Whatever you're dealing with, if accompanied by substantial feelings, as well as whether it's favorable or unfavorable, makes an in-depth perception of your subconscious.

Brainstorming is one of the ideal solutions when an issue arises. An additional approach to the trouble resolving is lateral thinking. The very first impulse when a problem emerges is to go straight to the heart of the matter for a remedy.

That does not always function, nonetheless. Occasionally, there doesn't appear to be a simple approach to the remedy. That's where the association of ideas is available. Allow's claim as an example, that you have a crucial client that you need to consult with ASAP.

You welcome him to your workplace, but he says he can not make it. What do you do? Sit down and also begin providing as many ideas as you can to make it feasible for the two of you to somehow satisfy and also review business. There is a symbol utilized in the association of ideas called Po.

This represents 'Provocative procedure.' It is used to recommend a suggestion which per se may not always be a good remedy; however, it assists in relocating your believing to a brand-new area, where you can explore some originalities, roll them around and also see just how they might offer the service to the problem.

For that reason, that customer does not wish to come to you. What's next?

- Po: Do you go to him?

- Po: How around a video conference?

- Po: Could you send out someone else in your place?

- Po: Exactly how about attempting to negotiate with him? Ask him what it would certainly require to obtain him to find.

- Po: You could wait up until he alters his mind.

I believe you understand concerning lateral thinking. It's all right to come up with what may seem to be horrendous suggestions, suggestions you know will certainly not function. It could exceptionally well cause ideas that will, which's what you're aiming for. And also, it does work; many huge firms have utilized this approach of brainstorming to excellent advantage and beautiful earnings.

Right-Brain/Left-Brain

Have you ever wondered whether you were right-brained or left-brained? That's very challenging to determine and probably really to restrict in terms of your mental ability. Pigeonholing yourself is not an excellent idea anyway.

By informing yourself that since you are systematic about certain things, you have to be an analytical thinker, you are limiting your possibilities.

You may be excellent at something imaginative, but will certainly never recognize it if you're as well restricting. Just because you like being innovative, does not imply you can not manage numbers like an accountant, if you pick to. Attempt not to limit your mind's capacities. When it comes to refining details, both fifty percent of your brain can do it directly in various methods. The dominant side is generally made use of to process info; however, the discovering can be enhanced if both parties are made use of in balance.

 This suggests you'll need to pump up your much less leading side, exercise it a little bit. Knowing how each fifty percent of your mind works will certainly assist you to understand how to create a balance between the two sides.

The Left Side

- Procedures information in a linear design. That implies that it takes items of details, lines them up, and after that puts them in a sensible series, then generates a conclusion. List production is what left-brained individuals like to do.

 They enjoy daily planning timetables, and they take terrific fulfillment in inspecting each product off the checklist as they accomplish it.

- It has no problem when it pertains to signs such as words, letters, and math notations. The left-brain person is at residence with linguistic and mathematical troubles.

- Verbal thinking has no difficulty with self-expression. The left-brained person can describe the problem in detail, offering a step-by-step solution.

- Take care of fact extra easily and also adjusts to different scenarios with more simplicity. Whatever their setting tosses at them, they can adapt to it more quickly.

The Right Side

- Processes much more arbitrarily, avoiding from thing to thing, leaping from topic to topic, more of a leapfrog strategy.

- Demands things to be more concrete. They require to see and also touch an object, as opposed to discussing it.

- Non-verbal reasoning. Has more difficulty revealing themselves in words and needs every little thing in writing.

- Not quickly versatile to their atmosphere. As opposed to change, they prefer to alter the atmosphere.

Nobody has fairly determined precisely why; however, the ideal hemisphere or appropriate brain controls the left side of our bodies, processing what we see with our left eye; and on the other hand, the left hemisphere or left-brain controls the appropriate side of our bodies as well as processes what we see with our proper eye.

Several believe that this is what identifies whether you are left-handed or right-handed; however, researchers inform us it is not associated in any way. Yet, nobody can explain why many more musicians have been left-handed.

If you are right-handed, felt confident it doesn't indicate you can't be imaginative, if you choose to be.

Once more, do not narrow your vision concerning yourself, telling yourself you are restricted due to the leading side of your brain. Learn to stabilize as well as utilize both parties to the finest benefit.

It will take some technique; however, you can learn to process info on both sides of your mind. The artistic kinds can discover to be more direct as well as the rational types can find to be much more arbitrary.

You will also experience four various brain wave states. These are Beta, Alpha, Theta, as well as Delta. When your brain is in the Beta state, you are wide-awake and also very sharp. This is when your mind does at its finest, but not creatively.

The Alpha state is a slower brain wave state as well as your creative thinking begins to move. Solutions start to present themselves throughout this state.

In the Theta state, you are entirely loosened up and also are concentrated much more on what's taking place within you.

You'll find this is remarkably similar to a reflective state as well as you might even uncover that the service to an issue comes to be extremely clear; you can see the 'broad view.'

When your brain is in the Delta state, you are sound asleep as well as it's time for your mind to charge, to get you ready for one more day and even more troubles and the requirement for imagination.

Though you are asleep, your mind is still working; indeed, it never quits; however, It does decrease enough that the chatter quits. While you're awake, your brain is making connections throughout the semantic network in a consistent circulation of information.

While you're asleep, nevertheless, your mind loses those links; it does, in reality, closed down for reenergizing. That's while you're in a deep sleep when the mind is dreaming, the links are still bending about in your account, much like it does when you're awake. Scientists think that the deep sleep cycle allows the cortical circuits to shut out the sound of the continuous links, to allow your mind to rest and also recuperate for the following day.

How To Keep The Brain Web Cam In Any Situation

We all have triggers that ignite our moods. Whether you have a sensitivity as a whole, tend to snap when you're stressed out, or snap when you get to a particular limitation, you have most likely spent a minimum of a long time wondering how you can keep one's cool in irritating situations.

 Besides, remaining calm isn't just vital for practical reasons (such as getting along in the work environment). It's additionally incredibly crucial for your total health, as tension is liked to an enhanced threat of a variety of illness.

Yet how do you keep your cool when somebody (or something) is pushing your switches? We'll check out a vast array of tricks and also methods that you can make use of in a variety of contexts, both in your professional as well as personal life.

 And when you find out exactly how to stay tranquil under pressure, mostly all of life's obstacles will be less complicated for you to conquer.

Why Do We Snap?

It is essential to give some believed to why and also exactly how you snap. This is various for everyone. We all interpret rage in a different way, and what drives you to diversion might not bother another person in any way.

Typically talking; however, one of the most usual triggers for temper consist of the following:

- A lack of control/feelings of powerlessness
- Really feeling threatened (physically or psychologically).
- Injustice or unfairness.
- Feeling unheard.

It may aid you in making a list of your triggers before going forward, as this can assist you in using the particular strategies we'll be clarifying. It's additionally worth keeping in mind that the things that make you upset are affected by your past experiences, as are the behaviors your exhibition in feedback to anger.

We over internalize ineffective messages when we're young, and also bringing them to aware recognition is the first step towards overcoming them.

Consider what your family, good friends, and teachers educated you concerning temper when you were maturing, either clearly or via their very own habits.

For instance, if you saw a lot of physical violence in your youth, you might fast to begin battles. On the other hand, if you saw moms and dads ingesting and also denying their temper as opposed to recognizing it, you may turn your rage inwards.

How To Keep One's Cool: Advice

In the face of anger or pain, our vanities are frequently all as well quick to react. However, ask on your own: when has your very own violence ever aided to solve a scenario, or to make you feel better? Really did not it just make you feel even worse?

When one more person is angry with us or sets out to injure us, the most vital thing to keep in mind is that every act is an act of love. When your companion utilizes restless words with you, you're put down or jeered at by a loved one or perhaps when that individual on the street shouts discriminative abuse at you; every one of these seeming acts of hatred was in reality, an act of love.

That's right; you read it right here; it is an act of love.

You see, whatever we do or claim or believe is in connection to something we love. So, when people do something hateful, this is, in fact, an outcome of their love for something, a desire they are incapable of connecting.

This leads us to exactly how we can best reply to somebody sharing anger. By far, the very best feedback is to ask a question, the concern being:

' What is hurting you?'
What is hurting that individual so severely that they feel they must harm you to heal? It is such a simple sentence, but it is one that ought to alter your entire point of view and also your life, right.
Asking a person this concern despite their anger works for a range of reasons. First off, by asking this inquiry, you lose your need to transform the thoughts or words of the other person.
This is what goes to the heart of the majority of conflicts: a requirement to reshape the point of views and ideas of the various other person.
 Nonetheless, by having a genuine problem of what may be harming this mad person, you're attesting to them that you acknowledge and approve their thoughts as well as their sights hold true for them.
Typically, having the ability to see through a person's craze and reveal a real rate of interest in what's taking place in their world can be enough to help them let go of their anger and also open up.
So, the initial idea on how to keep one's cool is to remember, following time you're challenged by anger, to ask that all-important inquiry: exactly how are you harming? It is as easy as that.

Keeping one's cool With Your Associates

Allow's start by considering just how to stay calm and also control your temper in the workplace. Three essential strategies will undoubtedly help you agree with coworkers, every one of which enables you to assert on your own appropriately while not only accepting disrespect or unfair therapy.

1. Don't Take It Personally

In many cases, disputes at the office will have practically absolutely nothing to do with you or the worth of your concepts. Instead, your colleague's ways of behaving, talking, as well as thinking is everything about them and their very own instabilities.

If you have a short-fused individuality, try to hold onto this reality whenever you start to feel outraged or upset. When you begin to feel angry at the office, ask on your own what needs your associate is meeting by taking care of you in this way.

You'll usually swiftly begin to see that their behavior all boils down to insecurity, a need to really feel crucial, and even jealousy.

2. Be The Voice Of Reason

A big part of learning how to keep one's cool at the office entails recasting on your own in a brand-new duty.

Rather than being the individual that is always pissed off, purposely calm yourself with deep breathing when somebody else's temper begins to increase. Speak clearly and also gradually, thinking of your words before utilizing them.

This type of reasonableness will certainly typically help to de-escalate the various other individuals, motivating them to pull back from their angry position.

As a benefit, if you do this commonly adequate after that, you'll obtain a track record for remaining rational in a crisis, which could certainly help your promotion prospects!

3. Take A Step Back

Taking a go back can do a great deal to control your mood. To put it, remove yourself from your position and try to take on a neutral, third-party point of view instead.

Check out the scenario you remain in, and also ask what will certainly occur if you shed your temper, begin shouting or react psychologically.

Usually, the lasting results won't benefit you, and also might include a requirement to say sorry later on (despite whether you were justified in accessing the very least rather angry). Consider this: will the critical things that are making you upset still make you angry this moment following year? If not, grit your teeth and also let it go this time.

How To Keep Calm With Your Pals

Trying to manage rage in your individual life can be more challenging than it is at work, as there is a more significant psychological, financial investment and even more liberty to speak your mind.

However, there's additionally a higher price if you can not keep one's cool, so attempt these three techniques to keep your social life on an even keel.

1. Maintain Viewpoint

First of all, reflect on whether it deserves making a big deal out of the problem that's causing a conflict with your pal.

Occasionally, it will be as well as will undoubtedly connect to the core of your partnership or a profound clash of values. Most of the time, however, the dispute may really feel essential in the moment yet most likely does not have longer-term importance.

Furthermore, a lot of conflicts with pals are based on misunderstandings and can be fixed by requesting for clearness. So, when you feel irritation rising, taking merely a few seconds to ask on your own "Does this issue to our friendship?" can stop you from producing a break.

2. Make A Joke

Wit is a widely known defense mechanism; however, when released properly, it can be a healthy and balanced one. Specifically, it can soothe a person with a short temper as well as can move your pal's focus back to your commonalities.

Indeed, you require to be cautious concerning what kind of remark you make as well as how you make it, yet a light referral to an in-joke or a pertinent, funny memory can do a whole lot to soothe stress.

And also, when you have chuckled together, you might locate that whatever was formerly causing the dissonance just doesn't appear so weighty anymore.

3. Consider What You Will indeed State

Choose your words meticulously when you're frustrated at a close friend. While you have every right to reveal discontent, an outburst of rage can do irreparable damages. Try to concentrate on uncontentious declarations that connect clear, details points about just how you feel. Mainly, utilize "I" declarations and stay clear of "always" and also "never ".

For example, "I feel disrespected by the fact you were an hour late" is a whole lot more likely to bring about an efficient resolution than "You're constantly so late, it's obvious you do not care regarding me in any way!".
Both statements enable you to get your sensations out, but the previous is reasonable while the latter is inflammatory.

How To Keep Calm With Your Family

Occasionally, members of the family can be the most different to handle, and discovering just how to keep one's cool in stressful scenarios revolves around recognizing that these individuals have a distinct capacity to irritate you up!

Try a mix of the adhering to three techniques.

1. Change Your Frame of mind

Your assumptions have a vast influence on exactly how you feel and behave during family member's occasions.

 As an example, if you enter presuming that your uncle is mosting likely to drive you insane, after that, you can bet he will! Instead, try to turn up for these celebrations with a calculated concentrate on the crucial things you're anticipating, the people you like most, and the high qualities you enjoy.

Mental research studies reveal that you truly can train your brain to act in this way which the a lot more you do it the far better able you are to concentrate on the positives without snapping.

2. Seek Common Ground

It's easy to obsess over all the worrying factors of disagreement; however, if you genuinely wish to keep your cool when you're with family members, then it's much more valuable to look for commonalities.

There are lots of points that you share, which is precisely why your mind is attracted to pick out the inconsistencies, to begin with!

Before (or throughout) a family member's event, attempt to remember specific areas where you, as well as your family members, remain in the arrangement. If things obtain stressfully, move the conversation in the direction of these topics.

 And also, also just keeping this common ground in mind can make you feel extra obliging and also receptive.

3. Breathe

It all else falls short and you're beginning to feel genuinely flustered, take a couple of minutes away from the team and calm yourself down before saying something you might regret. As soon as you're alone, attempt breathing in for a count of 10, and afterward out for a matter of ten.

Each of these sluggish, deep breaths will undoubtedly slow your heart rate and tell your body that there's nothing to be emphasized around.

If you can't find a hassle-free reason to get on another room, even a quick restroom break will undoubtedly give you a possibility to obtain your mood back under control.

keeping Calmness With Your Partner

Lastly, it is necessary to recognize the specific stress factors that come as part of any charming long-term relationship. When points get severe with your partner, look to one of these techniques to find a resolution.

1. Acknowledge Your Limitations

Every person has restrictions on their tolerance, and also it's vital to discover how to acknowledge you're not in the best headspace to settle an argument. When you sense that you're too mad or dismayed to give ground, you usually come to be less practical and also extra defensive.

At this moment, it's handy to state something like, "I do want to function this out with you, but I require some time to myself to cool down before I can talk with you properly.

" This is better than merely leaving, which can leave your companion troubled as well as might inadvertently indicate that you have to rate of interest in comprising.

2. Take Charge

If a minimum of one of you knows how to obtain their temper controlled, debates in between you are a lot less most likely to rise to the level of fury. If you want your partner to cool down, you require to show a level of calmness yourself.

So, keep your voice degree, take possession of your very own feelings, select your words carefully, and do not deploy disrespects that are created to hurt your companion. Nonetheless, as you do this, beware not to dip into natural aggressiveness instead of calmness. To put it, don't try to share a sense of supremacy or suggest that your partners show immaturity.

3. Be Prepared To Concession

Ultimately, the ability to the concession is just one of the main points that aids to suffer a happy connection. When you are at disparity with your partner, try to advise yourself that you ought to be interacting to discover a solution that meets at least a few of both of your needs.

 This is a lot more effective way of thinking than the competitive strategy that focuses on "winning".

In a lot of cases, even claiming this out loud can assist you both remain tranquil. While truthfully expressing your feelings, you can also note that you prepare as well as going to endanger which your partner's happiness matters a great deal.

Do you occasionally really feel that there's so much extra you could do with your smarts, only something is continually holding you back, be it mind haze, the lure of the Net, or another thing ultimately? Chances are, you're not the only one: The market is including attractive guide-books for brain-owners. So why should you read this publication summary?

Initially, they're sincere: They do not promise you'll come to be the next Einstein in a couple of weeks.

Second, unlike other programs, this book summary does not need you to stop your day job and center your whole life around your new mind workouts. Instead, you'll discover simple, functional suggestions that assist you in making the best of the bad brain you have-- with just a few small lifestyle changes, like consuming a lot more berries.

Third, all the advice you'll discover is based upon solid science.

And also lastly, it's a fast and enjoyable read.

In this recap of Activate Your Brain by Scott G. Halford, you'll find out.

- why we're not all that various from chimpanzees;

- why back puts can improve the performance of a basketball team; and.

- how jogging can help your mind fixing itself.

The Thalamus and Hypothalamus

Both the thalamus and also hypothalamus are related to changes in emotional reactivity. The thalamus, which is a sensory "way-station" for the remainder of the brain, is most crucial as a result of its links with various other limbic-system frameworks.

The hypothalamus is a small part of the mind located just below the thalamus on both sides of the 3rd ventricle.

Sores of the hypothalamus disrupt numerous unconscious functions (such as respiration and also metabolic process) and some so-called inspired behaviors like sexuality, combativeness, and cravings.

The side parts of the hypothalamus appear to be entailed with satisfaction and craze, while the medial part is linked to aversion, annoyance, and a tendency for irrepressible and also loud giggling.

The Cingulate GyrusThe cingulate gyrus is located on the medial side of the mind next to the corpus callosum. There is a whole lot to be discovered this gyrus, but it is understood that its frontal component web links smell and views with pleasant memories of previous emotions. This region likewise takes part in our emotional response to pain as well as in the law of hostile habits.

The Basic Ganglia

The primary ganglia are a group of cores lying deep in the subcortical white matter of the frontal wattles that organizes motor habits. The caudate, putamen, and also globus pallidus are significant parts of the basal ganglia. The primary ganglia appear to act as a gating mechanism for physical motions, hindering potential moves till they are appropriate for the scenarios in which they are to be executed. The primary ganglia are also entailed with:

- rule-based practice understanding (e.g., launching, quitting, monitoring, temporal sequencing, as well as keeping the suitable motion);.
- preventing unwanted activities and also allowing desired ones.
- picking from potential activities.
- electric motor preparation.
- sequencing.
- predictive control.
- functioning memory.

- interest.

Neuroplasticity

Neuroplasticity is the mind's capacity to develop brand-new neural pathways to account for discovering and also the procurement of new experiences.

The brain is regularly adjusting throughout a lifetime, though sometimes over the essential, genetically figured out amount of times. Neuroplasticity is the mind's capacity to produce brand-new neural pathways based upon brand-new experiences.

It describes changes in neural paths and also synapses that result from modifications in habits, environmental as well as neural processes, and alterations resulting from physical injury.

Neuroplasticity has replaced the previously held theory that the brain is a physiologically static body organ, and discovers just how the mind adjustments throughout life.

Neuroplasticity happens on a selection of levels, ranging from little cellular modifications arising from learning to significant cortical remapping in feedback to injury.

The role of neuroplasticity is extensively recognized in good advancement, finding out, memory, and also recovery from brain damage.

During a lot of the 20th century, the agreement amongst neuroscientists was that mind structure is fairly unalterable after a critical period throughout very early youth.

It holds that the mind is especially" plastic" throughout childhood years' critical period, with brand-new neural connections creating regularly.

Nevertheless, current findings reveal that several facets of the mind stay plastic also right into adult.

Plasticity can be demonstrated throughout practically any knowing. For one to bear in mind experience, the wiring of the mind should change.

Discovering happens when there is either an adjustment in the internal framework of neurons or an enhanced number of synapses between neurons.

Researches performed utilizing rats highlight how the brain modifications in action to experience: rats that resided in extra enriched settings had bigger nerve cells, even more DNA and RNA, larger cortexes, and more abundant synapses contrasted to rats who lived in sparse environments.

An unusual effect of neuroplasticity is that the mind task associated with a given feature can move to a different place; this can arise from everyday experience, and also occurs in the process of healing from mental injury.

Neuroplasticity is the basis of goal-directed experiential restorative programs in rehabilitation after brain injury.

For instance, after an individual is blinded in one eye, the part of the mind associated with processing input from that eye doesn't just sit idle; it handles brand-new features, possibly processing aesthetic data from the remaining eye or doing another thing entirely.

This is because while some parts of the brain have a regular feature, the brain can be "rewired"-- all due to plasticity.

Synaptic Trimming

" Synaptic (or neuronal or axon) trimming" describes neurological regulatory procedures that promote changes in the neural framework by lowering the total number of neurons as well as synapses, leaving other reliable synaptic arrangements. At birth, there are about 2,500 synapses in the cortex of a human infant. By three years old, the cortex has about 15,000 synapses. Because the baby mind has such a significant ability for growth, it has to eventually be pruned to get rid of unnecessary neuronal frameworks from the account.

This procedure of pruning is referred to as apoptosis or set cell death. As the human brain creates, the need for much more intricate neuronal organizations comes to be much more significant, as well as less complex associations formed at youth are replaced by more delicately interconnected frameworks.

Pruning eliminates axons from synaptic links that are not functionally appropriate. This process reinforces essential connections and removes weaker ones, developing a lot more efficient neural interaction.

Generally, the variety of neurons in the cerebral cortex boosts until adolescence. Apoptosis takes place throughout very early youth and teenage years, after which there is a decline in the variety of synapses.

About 50% of neurons present at birth do not endure until the adult years. The choice of the trimmed neurons follows the "utilize it or lose it" principle, implying that synapses that are frequently utilized have stable connections, while the rarely used synapses are gotten rid of.

Disclaimer

This book is not intended as a substitute for the medical advice of physicians. The reader should regularly consult a physician in matters relating to his/her health and particularly with respect to any symptoms that may require diagnosis or medical attention. (health, Brain)

about The Author

MY NAME IS Richard L Bolton
I really love educating people on how to stay healthy and live the life of their dreams.

Do Not Go Yet; One Last Thing To Do

If you enjoyed this book or found it useful, I'd be very grateful if you'd post a short review on Amazon. Your support does make a difference, and I read all the reviews personally so I can get your feedback and make this book even better.

Thanks again for your support!

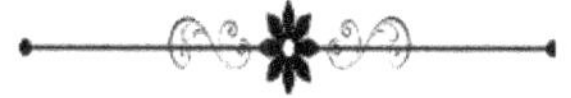